HEALING SPACES

HEALING SPACES

THE SCIENCE OF PLACE
AND WELL-BEING

Esther M. Sternberg, M.D.

THE BELKNAP PRESS OF
HARVARD UNIVERSITY PRESS
Cambridge, Massachusetts
London, England

Copyright © 2009 by Esther M. Sternberg
All rights reserved
Printed in the United States of America

First Harvard University Press paperback edition, 2010

Library of Congress Cataloging-in-Publication Data
Sternberg, Esther M.
Healing spaces : the science of place and well-being / Esther M. Sternberg.
p.   cm.
Includes bibliographical references and index.
ISBN 978-0-674-03336-8 (cloth: alk. paper)
ISBN 978-0-674-05748-7 (pbk.)
1. Architectural design—Health aspects.   I. Title.

RA770.S74 2009
725'.51—dc22   2009001734

To Penny and Dan, with love

CONTENTS

1

HEALING PLACES

There is a turning point in the course of healing when you go from the dark side to the light, when your interest in the world revives and when despair gives way to hope. As you lie in bed, you suddenly notice the dappled sunlight on the blinds and no longer turn your head and shield your eyes. You become aware of birdsong outside the window and the soothing whir of the ventilation system down the hall. You no longer dread the effort needed to get up, but take your first cautious steps, like a child, to explore the newfound space around you. The smell of food does not bring on waves of nausea or revulsion, but triggers hunger and a desire to eat. The bed sheets feel cool and soothing—their touch no longer sends shivers through you, like chalk-squeak on a blackboard. Instead of shrinking from others, you welcome the chit-chat of the nurse who enters the room.

This is the point when the destructive forces of illness give way to healing. In every sense, it is a turning point—a turning of your mind's awareness from a focus on your inner self to a focus on the outer world. Physicians and nurses know that a patient's sudden interest in external things is the first sign that healing has begun. But do our surroundings, in turn, have an effect on us? Can the spaces around us help us to heal? Can we design places so as to enhance their healing properties? And if we ignore the qualities of physical context, could we inadvertently slow the healing process and make illness worse?

The idea that physical space might contribute to healing

does, it turns out, have a scientific basis. The first study to tackle this question, published in *Science* magazine in 1984, showed that when hospital rooms have windows looking out on the natural world, patients heal more rapidly.

The sun was setting over Buzzard's Bay as the conference participants gathered for the evening. The sky glowed so brilliantly that even the white wine in their plastic cups seemed to catch fire.

"Look at that. That's got to have a healing effect!" Roger Ulrich waved his hand over the scene—dozens of sailboats moored in a still and fiery sea. He was standing on a bluff overlooking the bay at the southern end of Cape Cod, in front of a rambling gray saltbox-style building: the retreat and conference center of the National Academy of Sciences. It was here in August 2002, near the old whaling village of Woods Hole, Massachusetts, that John Eberhard, director of research at the American Institute of Architects (AIA), was hosting a collaborative workshop for scientists and architects, to explore the interface between architecture and neuroscience. It was the first workshop of what would become the Academy of Neuroscience for Architecture.

Ulrich's relaxed demeanor and boyish face belied the fact that he was a noted authority on the subject. He wasn't making an offhand remark or a haphazard guess. It was he who had performed the landmark 1984 study showing that window views could affect healing. He was responding to a question about what had inspired him to conduct that study.

"It just seemed like common sense," he said. "And the patients were already there, already being monitored for all sorts of things—heart rate, EKG, blood pressure, temperature—everything you could imagine. So we used those numbers to measure whether or not the windows had an effect on healing. We did it. And it worked."

He had examined the hospital records of patients who had undergone gall bladder surgery in a suburban Pennsylvania hospital during the period 1972–1981. He'd chosen forty-six patients, thirty women and sixteen men, whose beds were near windows that overlooked either a grove of trees or a brick wall. Twenty-three beds had views of nature and twenty-three did not.

Ulrich had recorded each patient's vital signs and other indicators of health, including dosages and types of pain medication and length of hospital stays. He'd found that patients whose beds were located beside windows with views of a small stand of trees left the hospital almost a full day sooner than those with views of a brick wall. Not only that, but the patients with nature views required fewer doses of moderate and strong pain medication. The results were dramatic and statistically significant. Ulrich had selected only forty-six patients to study because he was controlling for variables that could affect recovery, such as age, sex, whether the patients were smokers, the nature of their previous hospitalizations, the year of their surgery, even the floor their room was on. Each pair of patients—view of nature, view of brick wall—had been cared for by the same nurses, so differences in nursing care could not account for the differences in speed of recovery. Even doubters had to sit up and take notice.

The notion that nature was important to healing had been around for thousands of years—going back to classical times, when temples to Asclepius, the Greek god of healing, were built far from towns, high up on hilltops overlooking the sea. But by the late twentieth century, state-of-the-art hospitals were generally designed to accommodate state-of-the-art equipment. The more scanners and X-ray devices a hospital had, the more electroencephalograms and electrocardiograms it conducted, and the more sophisticated its biochemical blood and urine tests, the more advanced its care was considered to be. Often, the hospital's physical space seemed meant to optimize care of the equipment rather than care of the patients. In the early 1970s, one could still find hospitals where the only department that was air-conditioned was the Radiology Department, because the delicate equipment could not tolerate the summer heat. As reliance on and awe of medical technology increased in the mid-twentieth century, the comfort of the patients was somehow pushed aside and their surroundings were often ignored. Hospital planners assumed that patients could adapt to the needs of technology, rather than the other way around. When did this happen? When did the focus change from the patients to the disease, from healing to diagnosing and treating?

In the nineteenth century, hospitals were built with large windows and even skylights. Although this was done for the sake of visibility, in the days before powerful electric-light sources had been perfected, it was also done to help patients heal. Clinics and hospitals were designed to take maximum advantage of available sunlight, with large windows facing south and a solarium at the end of each ward. Even the word "solarium," meaning a room where patients could sit and absorb the healthful rays of natural light, is derived from *sol,* the Latin word for "sun."

In the late nineteenth and early twentieth centuries, the notion that sunlight could heal was very much in vogue. The great scourges in those days, before the development of antibiotics, were infectious diseases, especially tuberculosis. Sunlight and open windows were thought to be among the most effective means of purifying the air. In 1860, Florence Nightingale wrote that darkened rooms were harmful and sunlit rooms healthful; large, airy, bright rooms were the hallmark of what came to be known as a "Florence Nightingale" hospital ward. In 1877, a paper was presented to the Royal Society in London showing that sunlight could kill bacteria. In 1903, Dr. Auguste Rollier opened a sunlight clinic in the Swiss Alps. This may have been an inspiration for Modernist architects of the 1920s and 1930s, who designed homes and hospitals to take advantage of the sun.

Roger Ulrich's 1984 study grew out of this tradition, but had an added twist. He wanted to test whether views of nature were calming, and whether, by reducing the stress of hospitalization, they could in turn improve health. His ideas were based on a long tradition in modern architecture that posited a connection between architecture, health, and nature. Prairie School architects like Frank Lloyd Wright and Modernists such as Richard Neutra and Alvar Aalto designed buildings that appeared to grow out of their natural settings. In Neutra's structures, the glass walls seemed to melt away, allowing the indoor space to merge, almost seamlessly, with the outdoors.

Both Aalto and Neutra were explicit about the health benefits of well-planned architecture and about the importance of nature and natural views in health and healing. This concept may have had its roots in the tuberculosis sanatoriums of the nineteenth and early twentieth centuries, in the days before antibiotics. Patients with TB were sent to hospitals high in the mountains, in the hopes that the air at those altitudes would snuff out the infection. A perhaps unintended advantage was that these hospitals were all located in beautiful and isolated natural settings.

Indeed, the TB sanatorium designed by Alvar Aalto, built in 1929–1932 in the town of Paimio in his native Finland, became the standard for all later hospitals. It featured a patients' wing with light-filled rooms that faced south and overlooked a pine forest. The resting lounge was also bright, with a wall of tall windows looking out on forest views. Aalto was careful to stipulate that the surroundings be pleasant and tranquil. He even designed the furniture with the patients' comfort in mind, slanting the back of his sleek, laminated-wood "Paimio" chairs so as to ease the patients' breathing.

Although Richard Neutra admired and emulated the way

Frank Lloyd Wright embedded buildings in natural surroundings, he went beyond Wright, using steel and concrete and walls of glass to create structures that had a much lighter and airier feel and that blended indoors with outdoors. His Lovell "Health House" in Los Angeles—designed for the physician and *Los Angeles Times* health-column writer Philip Lovell and his wife, Lea—fit with the couple's convictions about health. It had views of nature on all sides.

These Modernist architects based their work on theories of the interface between design and health, but Roger Ulrich was the first to actually measure the effects of patients' surroundings on the healing process. The question at the Woods Hole Conference was not so much *whether* windows and nature views could heal, but *how* the healing mechanism operated. What brain pathways did windows and their views of nature activate? And how might these affect the immune system and its healing process?

John Eberhard, in his late seventies at the time of the conference, was a complicated man. He had held many important posts, including the chair of the Department of Architecture at Carnegie Mellon University. He had come up through the ranks in an era when architecture was almost exclusively the purview of white Protestant men. It had been a time when even the now world-famous architect Frank Gehry was persuaded by his wife to change his birth name, Goldberg, in order to get ahead. Perhaps because of his life experience, Eberhard wore his authority on his sleeve. He was a man used to wielding power and getting results, fast, and he sometimes pushed underlings almost to the point of tears to get things done. But under this tough exterior he had a softer side. He could come close to tears when talking about his legacy and his vision for his beloved field of architecture. He was also a talented artist who could execute quick, detailed sketches of buildings. And he read voraciously in pursuit of his interests, especially, at this juncture, in the field of neuro-science.

In 2002, Eberhard's title as director of research at the American Institute of Architects was a bit of an oxymoron, since the AIA was at times ambivalent about its role in research. Its primary mission is to set and maintain the highest standards in architecture, not to oversee or support research. But the AIA governance structure charged its CEO with setting programmatic priorities for its "knowledge communities," including architecture of hospitals, churches, schools, technology, and building science. Norman Koonce, a gracious, erudite gentleman from Lousiana, was then CEO and had long been interested in how architecture could enrich the human experience. In fact, he had recruited Eberhard in part with this goal in mind. The interface between architecture and neuroscience fit perfectly with these goals, and Koonce gladly supported exploring how the fields could inform one another. The workshop at Woods Hole brought together architects, neuroscientists, and psychologists whose expertise spanned the areas of stress research, visual perception, and environmental psychology.

If they could understand how physical surroundings affect emotions and how emotional responses to architecture affect health, then people's health could be taken into account in the design of buildings. Perhaps architects might even have some objective ammunition when trying to convince clients to spend a little more on larger windows and natural settings. Perhaps "green" design would turn out to be as beneficial to individuals' health as it is to the planet's health.

In his 1954 book *Survival through Design,* Richard Neutra said: "A workable understanding of how our psychosomatic organism ticks, information on sensory clues which wind its gorgeous clockwork or switch it this way or that, undoubtedly will someday belong in the designer's mental tool chest." In those days, the tools of neuroscience and immunology had not yet advanced to the point where they could be included in that tool chest. Today they have. And this is what the Woods Hole conference was all about: how to use those tools to inform the fields of neuroscience and architecture, and in turn promote healing.

The decision to include environmental psychologists like Roger Ulrich represented something of a rapprochement among the fields represented at the workshop. For decades, psychologists had been studying the effects of physical space on various aspects of mood, problem solving, and productivity. But as often happened in the scientific community, their methods, based in large part on participants' responses to questionnaires, were viewed by more biologically oriented investigators as "soft science." For their part, the architects had long known about these findings and felt there was nothing new to be learned from this approach. Nonetheless, the workshop provided a forum for a rich exchange of ideas—a chance for each field to contribute to the exploration of how the brain responds to built space, and how physical context in turn could foster good health, productive energy, and creative thought.

At Woods Hole, after a series of introductory lectures, the conferees broke up into working groups, each co-chaired by a neuroscientist and an architect. Roger Ulrich chaired the "Windows" group. These smaller sessions were meant for brainstorming. The "Windows" group would use the time to speculate freely about how windows might promote healing, and also to come up with ideas about what each discipline could measure. Why and how could window views affect healing? Was it because they provided more natural light? More airflow? Access to the sounds and smells of nature? Awareness of the rhythms of day and night? Did they simply distract patients from the monotony of days trapped in bed?

The architects in the group went first. They could measure

light intensity, wavelength, and color; temperature; airflow; and levels of activity in the scene being viewed. They went through the list of all the qualities that one could measure with sophisticated instruments in minute detail, to quantify every imaginable characteristic of physical space. This list would make it possible to design a study where researchers could measure and control these variables, in order to work out which factor or factors might explain the windows' effects.

The neuroscientists went next. They could monitor areas in the brain that became active when the patient was looking at a scene. They could measure physiological responses such as stress and relaxation. They could measure stress hormones in saliva, and changes in heart-rate variability and breathing. And they could measure general indicators of health such as immune responses, dosages of pain medications prescribed, and length of hospital stays.

The group concluded that by combining the most advanced tools of neuroscience, architecture, and engineering, one could dissect and measure each feature of a patient's physical environment, and the way each of those stimuli was received by the patient's brain and body. Researchers might then be able to identify elements in the physical environment that help people heal.

But could all this really be done? Would it be possible to isolate the single or several factors in the physical environment that contribute to healing? Or would it turn out to be something more—something intangible—that makes some places heal and others harm? Perhaps the most important thing a window does is provide a portal—an escape from the frightening, painful reality of disease, or a way of accessing memories of a better time and place. Maybe windows exert their effect by allowing a patient to step into a space of meditation—a reverie that brings not just distraction but relief. And relief could bring healing, through all those beneficial chemicals that flow from the brain through the body and change illness into wellness. Any or all of these hypotheses were possible, the workshop concluded. Research would confirm which ones were valid.

The conferees at Woods Hole were by no means the only ones advocating a collaboration between neuroscience and architecture to answer these questions. A new field does not emerge solely from the efforts of a few individuals, though it certainly needs individuals with vision, courage, perseverance, and drive to build and sustain it. A new field emerges after years, often decades, of accumulated knowledge, which at some point takes off exponentially. But even this often stems from thousands of years of implicit knowledge and questions that have been circulating in the general culture.

The idea that built space may affect health could not be investigated in scientific terms without the late twentieth-century advances which established that connections between the brain and the immune system are essential to maintaining health. Implicit in an understanding of the mind-body connection is an assumption that physical places that set the mind at ease can contribute to well-being, and those that trouble the emotions might foster illness. It would take significant advances—elucidating how the brain perceives physical space, how we remember and navigate the world around us, and how all this can affect emotions—to lay the groundwork for a new field linking those who design physical space with those who seek to understand the brain's responses to it. Collaborative intellectual endeavors between neuroscientists and architects are not new. From the days when scientists first began to study the brain, architects played a prominent role in attempts to map the brain and its mysterious structures.

Some four hundred stone steps lead up through the dome of St. Paul's Cathedral, built four centuries ago in London by the architect Sir Christopher Wren. Climb those steps and you will come to a narrow balcony ringing the dome's interior, halfway to the top. It is called the Whispering Gallery because two people can stand at opposite sides of the enormous space and carry on a conversation in whispers, every word clearly intelligible. Children who visit the dome delight in trying out the acoustics.

But Wren didn't build St. Paul's so that people could play games. He built it, and many other churches in the vicinity—a "flock of Wrens," Londoners call them—to replace structures destroyed in the Great Fire of 1666. If you wander into the cathedral when the choir is practicing, you might hear the crystalline voice of a countertenor wafting up past the Whispering Gallery to the very top of the dome—a voice so clear that no matter where you stand, it seems the singer is standing next to you, and this with no microphones or amplification. You feel a sense of awe and peace in that vast space, exactly as Wren had intended when he built the dome.

Walk west from St. Paul's, past the staid stone buildings that house the courts and legal offices of Temple Bar, and soon you come to Oxford Street's bustling shopping district. Your gaze is attracted by windows filled with goods from all over the world. Keep walking down Oxford Street past Oxford Circus, make a little jog to Cavendish Square, and you reach the Royal Society of Medicine, part of the Royal Society established around the same time that Wren built his cathedral. One of the society's founders was Sir Thomas Willis, the anatomist whose intricate drawings of the brain, published in 1664, first showed what that organ really looked like. Before Willis opened up cadavers' skulls and dissected the contents, physicians and scientists had little notion of what the brain looked like, much less of what it did. Today, medical students know his name because it remains associated with the ring of nutritive blood vessels at the base of the brain—the "Circle of Willis." This group of arteries looks unim-

portant, but the rupture of a single one will cause almost instant
death, because the vessels are so close to the brain regions that
support the vital organs.

It was anatomical knowledge such as this that helped to shape
the modern era of medicine—the understanding that abnormal-
ities of anatomy could lead to disease. To discover this principle,
anatomists first had to map human anatomy accurately. They did
so by dissecting corpses (often stolen from graveyards) and carefully drawing what they saw. The only tools they had for gaining
entry into the skull were hacksaws, hammers, and chisels. And
once inside, all they could use to dissect the delicate brain tissue
were primitive knives, scissors, and tweezers. Yet Willis was able
to produce drawings so detailed, so precise, so finely engraved,
that they could still be used today as a guide to every nook and
cranny of the brain.

Willis' treatise *Cerebri Anatome,* which so changed medicine,
presents drawings of the brain from all angles: above and below,
front and back and side, and slices all the way through. The illus-
trations—sharply engraved, and printed on fold-out leaves of
thick rag paper—alternate with pages of Latin text. If you visit
the library of the Royal Society of Medicine, you can request the
volume and, wearing white cotton gloves, page through it at
your leisure. Turn to the front of the book and you will make an
amazing discovery. Willis dedicated it, in Latin, to one of its il-
lustrators: Sir Christopher Wren.

Willis and Wren were friends and colleagues. In those days,
scholars didn't stay within the confines of their disciplines, but
often drifted into other areas of expertise. Wren had started off
as an anatomist, fascinated by the structures of the human body.
Only later did he find his calling as an architect. Indeed, there
are many similarities between the practice of architecture and
that of anatomy. Both require an ability to visualize a structure
in three-dimensional space and to render it in two dimensions,

on paper, so that those less skilled at visualization can see it as well. Both require an ability to rotate objects in one's imagination, to slice them and examine them in many planes. It must have been for this reason that Willis turned to Wren, an architect, when he needed help drawing what he saw.

Wren himself had unusual skill at dissection, as well as an inventive mind. He had helped to develop a technique of injecting ink into arteries, in order to trace blood flow. Together, Willis and Wren injected, cut, and teased apart vessels from brain tissue to clearly distinguish each tiny structure and allow Wren's artistic hand to render it on paper.

At the time these artist-scientists lived, it was impossible to say how the organ inside the skull could possibly affect thinking and feeling. Yet they had an inkling of the central role the brain played in these activities. About twenty years before the publication of *Cerebri Anatome,* the French philosopher René Descartes had drawn a rough sketch linking an object viewed to the viewer's eye and, through the brain, to movement of the arm. That sketch may have been the first to show explicitly that the brain receives sensory input from the environment and then, in some mysterious manner, makes us act.

Today, four centuries after Descartes made his rudimentary drawing and Christopher Wren designed his magnificent cathedral and illustrated Sir Thomas Willis' book, we can actually see, with the tools of modern science, how our sensory organs receive signals from the world around us, and how the cells and molecules of the brain work together to blend these signals into a perception, enabling us to sense and negotiate the spaces around us. We can discern how the nerve chemicals produced by the brain when we react to our environment may in turn influence the immune system that helps us heal. We can do all this without ever breaking through the skull.

With modern imaging tools we can slice the brain from every

possible angle without touching it, using instruments that detect magnetic fields or radiation or light. We can see how different parts of the brain work together, how the centers that produce and control our emotions interact with those parts that create thought and memory. With the modern techniques of biochemistry, cell biology, and molecular biology, we can piece together how the elements of the world around us, which we perceive through our senses, can trigger different areas of the brain in order to generate feelings of awe or fear or peace and comfort. We can understand, too, how these different kinds of emotions, when blended together, can promote healing.

We can use these new technologies to prove that the spaces through which we move—the contexts of our world—play a very important part in cementing memories. And we can measure how molecules of the immune system that are released when we are sick change our ability to form memories of place and space. We can show how these molecules change our moods, especially when we are sick. And finally we can show how, when we reencounter a place that evokes a certain mood, an emotional memory can revive in full force and change the brain's hormones and nerve chemicals to help or hinder healing.

In order to understand how this happens, we need to know both what healing is and what place is. If illness and health are nouns, then healing is a verb. It is movement in a desired direction—a journey that takes you from illness to health. There are as many kinds of healing as there are cells and organs in the body and diseases that can affect them, but all involve restoring the body to a state of balance. In fact, healing is going on all the time—microscopic bits of healing, at every moment of the day. The very fact that we are living means that we are being buffeted about, injured with every action we take and every stimulus to which we are exposed. Failure to heal after each insult would eventually result in death. It's like walking up a down escalator.

You must keep taking a step up in order to remain in the same spot. Health is that spot, and healing is the perpetual march you must make to stay there.

Healing also takes place in different regions of the body. It is easy to imagine a diseased liver or heart or lungs—filled with scar tissue or fatty deposits or infectious pus—going from illness to health. Gradually the infection clears, the fat dissolves, the scar shrinks, and the organ is restored to full functioning. What about the brain? It too can be filled with tumor cells, or clots, or inflammation, and some of these likewise can resolve. There are also illnesses of the mind—of our thoughts and our emotions. These can heal as well. In this kind of healing, brain chemicals and the cells that make them must find their right balance.

How a thought or an emotion emerges from those cells and brain chemicals is a process we do not yet understand. What we do know is that the same nerve chemicals and cell processes that create mood and imbalances of mood are also involved in our perception of the world around us. We construct an image of a place based on the information we receive through our senses, and somehow, somewhere—actually in many places in the brain—it all gets put together to create our sense of place. Just as healing is a constant process, so is sense of place. Our perception of place changes not only with our location, the weather, and the time of day—the physical elements of space— but also with our moods and our health. Our sense of where we are is continually being created and re-created in our brain, depending on current conditions and on our memories of what went on there.

Think of a widow, long married and recently bereaved. She finds herself in a resort town where she used to come year after year with her husband when he was well. His declining health prevented them from visiting here in the waning years of his life, and months of grieving have prevented her from coming back until now, a year after his death. She longs to revisit a tiny restaurant, not more than a hole in the wall where only the locals dined, which she and her husband had made their own. Night after night they used to come to the place for a simple supper— large prawns broiled in special spices were his favorite. They had a favorite waiter, too, who always chose the freshest seafood and showed it to them, before asking the chef to prepare it exactly as they liked. The place is not close to where she is staying now, but she had to go there, drawn by the memories and the desire to relive those days. She can't remember exactly where the restaurant is, since they always went on foot from their hotel. Now, as the cab winds its way through the dark and narrow streets, she recognizes the neighborhood, and, with a mixture of excitement and anxiety, finally sees the restaurant's awning and the pool of light spilling into the street. There's no window, not even a door, just an open wall, and, separating the tiny room from the street, a refrigerated glass case filled with fish, crabs, prawns, and octopus freshly caught from the bay. With trepidation she gets out of the taxi and walks up to greet the waiter, *their* waiter, who immediately recognizes her. In the same instant, he notices that her husband is not with her. They embrace, shed a few tears, recall his booming presence and the sadness of their loss. The waiter seats her at the couple's favorite table. She looks around and is flooded with emotions—happy memories of their times there together, mingled with sad ones of the present. The light, the smells, the sounds are all the same. One moment, she travels back into memory and revels in it; the next moment, she becomes aware of her husband's absence, and weeps. But there is something comforting about visiting this place one more time. The welter of emotions inside her is helping to close the wound and bringing her back to the stream of life.

It is at this level—in the brain and in the mind—that healing and places intertwine. Healing has a rhythm and a flow. Some illnesses stop and start, some have a downward course, and some resolve. The pace toward recovery is often agonizingly slow and often jerky, as sudden improvements alternate with backward steps. Imagine what one of Roger Ulrich's gall bladder patients must have experienced before waking up in that hospital bed by the window.

In the operating room, the surgeon, under the glare of the surgical lamp, swiftly and carefully put scalpel to skin. With one firm stroke the blade cut through the top layer of skin, through the underlying layer of yellow-white fat, down to the abdominal muscle. With another stroke the blade cut through the muscle, exposing the abdominal cavity just above the liver. In the early 1980s, when Ulrich performed his study, the incision would have been several inches long, exposing the liver's glistening reddish-brown surface. Today, it would be less than an inch, just enough to insert an optical device—a magnifying camera—through which the surgeon can peer. Once the gall bladder, like a green balloon filled with pebbles, is snipped from its stalk and removed, the surgeon works back up through layers of muscle, fat, and skin to suture the incisions.

These few cuts immediately set in motion a series of events that turn the body's energies toward a single goal: healing the wounds. The repair process is messy at best, and messier still if complications like infection arise.

It is the immune system that provides the machinery of healing. Many different kinds of immune cells, each with its special task, arrive on the scene like well-choreographed actors who know their cues and their places onstage. When the surgeon's blade pierces the skin and the tissue underneath, it also cuts through blood vessels. Sharp and clean as those cuts are, they inevitably kill cells as they rend the connections that hold together the surface of the skin. When cells die they release their contents, including chemicals that call living cells to the site. The cells they summon—white blood cells shaped like irregular spheres, called *monocytes*—have been happily floating through the bloodstream. Now they begin to assume a different shape, and no longer float smoothly through the blood but collide with the inner surface of the vessels. As they roll and bump along, they produce proteins on their surface that make them stick to the blood vessel walls. And then, like some primordial fish taking its first tentative steps onto land, they change shape even more. Bits of their surface reach out, like feet, and they begin to crawl and ooze, first along the blood vessel and then through cracks between the cells that make up the vessel's lining. They use these foot-like extensions, called *pseudopods,* to crawl through the tissues beneath the blood vessel, toward the wound, drawn inexorably by the scent of the chemicals released by the dying cells.

The substances that draw these cells toward them are proteins called *chemokines*—from the Greek words meaning "chemical" and "kinetic," literally "chemicals that make cells move." These molecules have an amazing power to summon cells that are crucial to the body's defense, the *phagocytes* (meaning "cells that eat"). These cells do indeed consume all of the foreign material in their path. Once a monocyte is activated and begins to move through the tissues, it is called a *macrophage* and begins to gorge itself with the debris it encounters. The feet on which it crawls reach out and engulf any dead or foreign tissue in its path. You can watch this drama in real time under a microscope, and even feed these cells tiny latex beads. They will envelop each bead until they swell to bursting. When they ingest dead or foreign material, they absorb it into pools of enzymes inside tiny balloons in their cytoplasm—the liquid inside the cell. These balloons are called *lysozomes,* and if their contents were to spill, the chemicals would destroy the nearby tissue. In fact, this is what happens when the surgeon's knife cuts through the cells. But when the enzymes are held safely inside a skin within a skin—inside the lysozome inside the macrophage—they become the cell's garbage disposal units. They quickly separate the debris into its component proteins, dismantle the proteins into bits and pieces, and then fragment the bits into the molecular building blocks (amino acids) that constitute those proteins. In this way the dead and dying tissues are broken down, recycled, and removed, making way for the next phase of healing.

New cells now stream into the site—cells whose job it is to fill the hole, to glue the edges of the cut together. These cells, called *fibroblasts,* make a kind of protein glue called *collagen.* This is what holds cells together in a matrix, to create the tissues—skin, tendon, fat, and muscle. It is what makes your skin firm and supple and elastic. And it is what creates a scar.

In the midst of all this activity, other cells arrive to fend off infection. These are *lymphocytes,* and there are many different kinds. They make antibodies, attack viruses, fend off bacteria. Each cell, while doing its job, also grows and divides, so that many more cells of each type accumulate at the scene, facilitating the healing process. It is this activity that causes the redness, heat, swelling, and pain at sites where healing is beginning. Only later does a scar appear.

All this takes a predictable amount of time. Even if you have very minor surgery—say, to remove a mole on your nose—you will be sent home with an instruction sheet that tells you when you can take off the outer pressure bandage (in twenty-four to forty-eight hours); when you can first wet your face or wash your hair (not before five to seven days); and when you should return to have the sutures removed (in seven to ten days). The reason doctors can foresee each step with such accuracy is that the healing process follows a set timeline.

The process is difficult to speed up, but it can be impeded—by drugs or infection or even stress. If your father has Alzheimer's disease and you are his main caregiver, you grieve every single day, over and over again. Here is the same man you've known throughout your life, but his body is now just a shell. As time goes on, relentlessly, you find less and less of his personality as you look into his face. You worry about his health, about his tendency to wander off, about his combative moments when he strikes out at those who try to help. You sleep poorly, in fits and starts, and you are tired every moment of the day. You are depressed and have lost your appetite. You are chronically stressed. All of this affects your immune system and its ability to heal.

Place, too, can have an effect on healing. If you are living in dark, cramped, crowded quarters where noise is constant, you will be stressed. If you are isolated, far from friends and family, you will be stressed. In such cases your immune system is burdened and the healing process slows. Wherever you are in the course of illness or healing, your physical surroundings can change the way you feel and, as a result, can change how quickly you heal. In all these contexts, communication between the brain and the immune system is vital. Besides bringing in new cells to help fight germs, molecules released by immune cells during infections also travel to the brain and change the way it functions. One of the things immune molecules do when we are sick is wipe out memory of our surroundings. The part of the brain that focuses on sensations from our inner organs becomes more active, and the part that focuses on the outer world shuts down. So we become exquisitely sensitive to internal signals from our throat or stomach or lungs, and acutely aware of every breath or twinge, and we lose interest in anything beyond the self.

The brain, in turn, sends its own signals to immune cells—hormones and nerve chemicals that can tune up or tune down the ability of immune cells to fight disease. There are many things that can influence the release of these chemical signals from the brain, and our surroundings play a very important part. How we perceive the world around us, its features of light and dark, sound and smell, temperature and touch, feed into the brain through all our senses and trigger the brain's emotional centers, which make us react. These emotional centers release nerve chemicals and hormones that can change how immune cells fight disease. In turn, through this communication, our awareness of space and place changes when we are ill, and changes yet again when we begin to heal.

We don't yet fully understand all the ways in which windows could affect healing. Their influence could stem from the light they provide, the colors one sees, the sounds one hears, the odors one smells. Or it might be due to a release from boredom, the escape they offer—or to some or all of these factors, depending on the individual's experience. But the remarkable thing is that the fields of neuroscience, immunology, psychology, architecture, and engineering have reached the point where scholars and practitioners are ready to talk to one another and learn from one another. In so doing, they will come closer to answering such questions about the effects of place on healing.

It was the immunologist and virologist Jonas Salk whose legacy brought together the experts at Woods Hole, through a request born of his own experience with the inspirational nature of a place. In the 1950s, while Salk was working to develop a polio vaccine in his basement laboratory in Pittsburgh, he came to an impasse. Frustrated and demoralized, he decided to take a sabbatical, and stayed for a time in the Italian town of Assisi. So inspired was he by the light and beauty and spiritual aura of the place, that he hit upon the solution to his problem. He rushed back to his lab and created his vaccine, which has since saved millions of lives.

Salk was never awarded the Nobel Prize, nor was he even admitted to the prestigious National Academy of Sciences. But he received a gift of land from the San Diego City Council, and enough money from the March of Dimes to build his own research center. Salk vowed that, in the spirit of Assisi, he would build the facility in a place suffused with light and surrounded by beautiful views—a place that would inspire the imagination of other scientists just as Assisi had inspired him. He chose La Jolla, near San Diego in Southern California, and worked with the architect Louis Kahn to build what many architects view as one of the greatest architectural achievements of the twentieth century: the Salk Institute.

Set atop the cliffs overlooking the Pacific Ocean, the institute comprises a pair of long, four-story buildings that stand perpendicular to the cliffs. They appear to be made of the same chalky stone as the cliffs, but in fact are made of concrete—a concrete that Kahn designed to resemble the native limestone. At Salk's request, every researcher is assigned not only lab space on the main floor, but also a private office on the second floor, overlooking the sea. The wood-paneled offices are quiet and peaceful—ideal spaces for contemplation. Between the two buildings is a travertine-paved promenade which blends in so well that the cliffs, the outdoor space, and the structures appear as a unified whole. The buildings are aligned so that the beams of the setting sun fall directly between them as it sinks beyond the sea. A narrow channel of water, running the length of the promenade and emptying into a reflecting pool, catches the sun's rays like fire. The institute is now a mecca for architects and scientists alike, and has become world famous for its research in basic science, molecular biology, and neuroscience.

When Salk came to Washington, D.C., in 1992 to accept the American Architectural Foundation's prestigious award for a building that has stood the test of time, he told the officers of the foundation about his experience in Assisi, which had led him to re-create with Kahn the same atmosphere on the La Jolla

cliffs. He recounted how it was Assisi and the spiritual experience of that place which had stirred his intuition and brought
him to his final breakthrough. He asked the architects to continue investigating the connection between architectural space
and creativity. This led to a series of gatherings at the Salk Institute to identify the power of architecture to enrich the human
experience. Salk hoped to foster links between scientists and architects so that researchers could capture and understand the atmosphere he had found so inspirational.

After Salk died, his request remained dormant in his will and
in the memory of those who'd been present at the foundation
award ceremony and subsequent gatherings. Then, in 2003, a
San Diego architect named Alison Whitelaw conceived an idea
that launched the Academy of Neuroscience for Architecture.

Whitelaw was at the forefront of sustainable design for public
facilities when she was elected president of the San Diego Architectural Foundation. She was familiar with the rich concentration of neuroscience research in the San Diego area—not only
at the Salk Institute, but also at the Scripps Clinic and Research
Institute, the University of California at San Diego, and the
Neurosciences Institute. As president she was charged with developing a "Legacy Project" for the next AIA national conference, to be held in San Diego the following autumn. Legacy
Projects sponsored by local AIA host chapters had often been
buildings designed and built by local architects, and they sometimes involved the establishment of foundations. When Whitelaw
heard of Salk's request from Norman Koonce, she decided that
rather than building a brick-and-mortar institute, she would establish a virtual edifice, one that would bring neuroscientists and
architects together to study the interface between their fields. As
luck would have it, Koonce, then president and CEO of the
American Architectural Foundation, had been at the 1992 award
dinner for Jonas Salk and at the many subsequent meetings
with him. When Whitelaw asked him for support, Koonce re-

called Salk's story of inspiration and his request that neuroscientists build an alliance with architects. He immediately put
Whitelaw in contact with John Eberhard, who was pursuing a
similar goal. The two joined forces to establish the Academy of
Neuroscience for Architecture in San Diego. This was the San
Diego Architectural Foundation's Legacy Project. With her quiet
demeanor and soft, British-accented voice, Whitelaw was an odd
partner for John Eberhard and his booming personality. But
their project, encouraged by the University of California and the
New School of Architecture in San Diego, attracted scientists
from all the major neuroscience research centers in the area,
along with architects from Southern California and around the
country. In his new position as CEO of the American Institute
of Architects, Koonce gladly backed the establishment of the
Academy of Neuroscience for Architecture. The idea had found
its home.

Though much research still needs to be done, the groundwork
has been laid. Each discipline is learning from the other. Only
with such knowledge can research move forward and new designs be conceived and implemented. Scientists have already
identified many features of the environment that affect our
brains and bodies and that contribute to healing. We can put
the puzzle together and understand how, as our senses absorb
stimuli from the spaces around us, different parts of the brain
become active and enable us to see and hear and touch and
smell. We can understand how sense perceptions trigger emotions that send molecules flowing through our bloodstream and
nerve cells. And we know how those molecules can affect the
immune system and its ability to heal. So we can truly begin to
understand how space and place, and something as simple as a
window with a view of trees, could turn the tide against illness
and speed the course of healing.

2

SEEING AND HEALING

If you were a patient in a hospital bed, just waking up from surgery, what would you prefer to see when you opened your eyes—a brick wall or a grove of trees? The choice seems obvious—or perhaps not. Perhaps you're a person who delights in counting rows of bricks and lines of mortar, in scanning surfaces for patterns, color variations, and flaws. But if Roger Ulrich's observations are correct, there is something about trees that promotes healing. Could it be their color—the soothing greens of nature? Could it be that trees provide more movement, more activity, more life to observe, so that you don't need to invent counting games to keep yourself occupied? Could it be the trees' shape that is calming and relaxing? Could it be that the light streaming through the window changes how you feel and how you heal?

At the second Woods Hole workshop on architecture and neuroscience, held in August 2004, Carla Shatz of Harvard Medical School's Department of Neurobiology was invited to advise because of her discoveries in vision science. If researchers were going to figure out how architectural space affects the brain, a neuroscientist with expertise in vision had to be involved. Shatz came to the workshop intrigued and a little skeptical, but with an open mind.

Her pedigree was impeccable. She had trained with Torsten Wiesel and David Hubel—two neuroscientists who'd shared the 1981 Nobel Prize in Medicine for their discovery that cells in the retina, and nerve cells in the parts of the brain that register vision, mainly respond to and detect edges—the contrast between light and dark. Hubel and Wiesel had implanted electrodes in the brains of cats, in the area that receives signals from the eyes: the visual cortex, at the back of the head. When they showed the cats a card marked with a single black stripe, the cats' visual cortex generated electrical activity in a line of nerve cells that matched the stripe. If they showed the cats a card with multiple stripes, the electrical activity likewise took the form of multiple stripes. The patterns were identical to each other, but the one in the brain was drawn in electrical impulses instead of shades of light and dark. Certain rows of nerve cells were switched on and certain rows were switched off, corresponding to the light and dark stripes each cat was shown.

Carla Shatz was a young Ph.D. student in neuroscience when she came to work with Hubel and Wiesel. She tackled the question of how it was that so many different kinds of cells, retinal cells and nerve cells, could maintain their spatial organization all the way from the back of the eye to the back of the brain—an arrangement that allowed those stripes of light and dark projected on the retina to be registered as stripes of on-and-off signals in the brain. Shatz made an important discovery: "cells that fire together wire together." During early development, nerve cells die if they receive no signals; they survive only when there is electrical activity. This activity establishes the circuits for the rest of an individual's life. And nerve cells maintain the same organization throughout an entire circuit.

Shatz was singularly creative, and was riveting when she talked about her passion for neuroscience. Her intellectual curiosity, meticulous scholarship, and contagious enthusiasm enabled her to rise quickly through the ranks to become the first woman chair of the Department of Neurobiology at Harvard Medical School. And she was among the first women to be elected president of the Society for Neuroscience—the most prestigious international body of neuroscience researchers, with a membership of approximately thirty thousand. At the Woods Hole workshop, Shatz's knowledge of the visual system was essential in the collaborative effort to understand how architectural space could affect the visual pathways in the brain, and thus how window views might influence healing.

When you look at an object, the light it reflects falls on the cells in the retina, which contain chemicals called pigments. Some of the cells, called *rods,* respond only to light and dark, while others, called *cones,* respond to different wavelengths of light—that is, to colors (rods and cones are named for their shape). When light hits the pigments in a retinal nerve cell, a chemical reaction occurs, triggering an electrical signal that travels along the cell's filamentous fibers (known as *axons*) until it reaches the ends of cells, where other chemicals are stored in little sacks. When the electrical impulse hits these vesicles, they empty their contents into the gulf between nerve cells. In this way, light is transformed into an electrical signal that jumps swiftly from one nerve cell to another and travels to many regions in the brain.

Bundles of these nerve fibers join together in a large cable-like structure called the *optic nerve.* Half of its fibers originate in the left eye and connect to the right side of the brain; those stemming from the right eye do the opposite. After relaying to a second nerve cell at a switching station in the brain stem, the electrical signals come to rest in the part of the brain that governs vision—the region at the back of the head called the *occipital lobe.* How do these electrical signals get translated into what you see?

Before you recognize an object, your eyes see bits and pieces of it—contrasting edges and lines. It is the visual cortex that puts these pieces together into a whole. If there is not enough information to make a continuous line, the brain connects the bits anyway, and you see a shape. Almost simultaneously, another part of the brain tries to match this picture to images stored in your memory. Whatever gives the closest match is the one you recognize. Then other parts of your brain recognize what it is and tell you what to do with it.

The brain is constantly scanning the objects in your visual field and matching them to images residing in your memory, the way a computer looks for a word when you click on the "search" function. When a match is found, the link lights up and we recognize what we see. The brain is a matching machine that stores memories and recognition of different types of objects in different places. Depending on the category in which your brain places the object, different parts of the brain become active—blood flow increases, nerve cells fire off electrical impulses, genes start making proteins, chemicals are released from nerve endings, and nerve cells signal to one another. You literally connect the dots and see the object.

When Roger Ulrich's patients looked out the window, was there something about the objects they saw that promoted or hindered healing? Perhaps the objects' shape, or their color, or how they were arranged? In order to answer these questions, we need to know exactly what an object is. Look at a hammer or a pair of eyeglasses (or at an image of them). You immediately know two facts: that they're not living creatures, and that you can use them to do something—pound a nail into a plank of wood, or improve vision. You know what the objects are, and also what they are not. You know that they are tools and that they are not animals. Look at a bird, or a picture of a bird, and you know right away that it's an animal and not a tool. Now look at the image of a hammer that has a head shaped like a bird, with a dot where you might expect to see an eye. You still know it's a hammer. But make the shaft of a hammer wider and rounder, perhaps even sketch in a couple of little legs, and your brain will recognize the object as a bird, even if the shape of the head is still hammer-like.

When you recognize the hammer as a tool, there's a spurt of electrical activity in the part of the brain that would become active if you were to use that tool. This region is the *motor cortex*, which governs movement in the muscles of your arm. It's as if you were preparing to use the hammer. But change the object just enough so that it looks like a bird—give the hammer-head eyes and make the prongs look like a beak—and the motor cortex gradually goes silent. A different part of the brain becomes active, the one that recognizes animals.

Each category of object that you see is recognized in a different place in the brain. Faces are recognized in one part of the brain, objects in another. Scientists know this because they can make images of functioning brains using techniques such as positron emission tomography (PET scans), magnetic resonance imaging (MRI scans), and computerized axial tomography (CAT scans); and when they image the brains of people who are being shown pictures of faces, the scans reveal activity in a tiny area of the temporal lobe called the *fusiform face area*. Patients who have had strokes or damage in this part of the brain can no longer recognize faces, though they can recognize other objects. In contrast, brain-damaged patients whose face area is intact can recognize faces but not other objects.

C.K., a twenty-seven-year-old man, sustained a closed-head injury when he was hit by a car while jogging. After he recovered from the accident, his ability to identify faces was above average, but only when pictures of the faces were displayed right-side up. When an image was upside down, C.K. couldn't recognize the face—and didn't even know he was looking at a face. And he had another bizarre problem. When he was offered a choice of foods at a cafeteria, he found the array frightening, since (as he said) all he could distinguish were colored "blobs." The blobs had to be identified for him before he could make a selection.

The Canadian researchers who studied C.K. in 1997 wanted to know if he could distinguish objects from faces. They showed him pictures inspired by the sixteenth-century Italian artist Arcimboldo, who created whimsical paintings from clumps of various objects such as fruits, vegetables, animals, or books. When C.K. was shown a series of faces composed in this way, he knew they were faces but was unable to recognize the constituent objects, seeing them simply as colored blobs. When pushed further to identify the objects, he could say only that in one case there seemed to be bags beneath the eyes—he did not recognize those bags as cherries. C.K.'s very selective impairment provides clear evidence that the part of the brain that recognizes faces is different from the part that recognizes objects.

Remarkably, there is even a brain region that specializes in recognizing buildings. Patients who have had strokes in this area often get lost because they can no longer recognize buildings as landmarks, even though they can identify other objects. In order to make up for their deficit, they navigate by using smaller features of their environment, such as doorknobs or benches. In brain-imaging studies of normal people, this small area displays an increase in nerve cell activity and blood flow when a person is shown a picture of a building, but remains unaltered when the person views a face or a car. It is hard to imagine why a particular brain region for building recognition might have evolved, especially since buildings appeared relatively recently in human evolution. Perhaps it evolved not for recognizing buildings per se, but for identifying large objects that can be viewed from a distance only from a limited number of angles—for example, hills or cliffs, which may have served as landmarks in a prehistoric landscape.

The brain's building-recognition area is just beneath another part of the brain called the *parahippocampal place area,* which recognizes scenes—that is, many objects grouped together. Some researchers have proposed that the brain uses large structures such as buildings to define the geometry of local space, and groups of smaller objects to identify a scene. Russell Epstein, a professor at the University of Pennsylvania, described the theory at another Academy of Neuroscience for Architecture workshop, this one, held in December 2003 in Washington, D.C., focused on healthcare facilities for the elderly. It explored the difficulties in visual perception that come with age—important information for architects designing spaces for elderly people.

Epstein described his work, in which he imaged the brains of volunteers as they were shown different kinds of pictures. He found that the parahippocampal place area became active when people viewed scenes, but was only weakly active when they viewed single objects and was not at all active when they viewed faces. In another study, he showed college students pictures of familiar and unfamiliar campuses and asked them to locate the places they viewed. Epstein found that recognizing familiar places and recognizing unfamiliar places involved two different parts of the brain. Memory was evidently important in locating a familiar scene but was not required for identifying an unfamiliar scene.

This phenomenon of recognition operates within us every day as we navigate our surroundings. Enter a department store from the parking lot. The store has many entrances that all look pretty much the same, so how do you find the one you want when it comes time to leave? You remember the things you saw in the department nearest the door through which you entered. Each item on display is recognized by your brain as an object—a watch, a scarf, a bottle of perfume. But in a grouping—jewelry, accessories, fragrances—they become part of the scene and a landmark for you when you want to find your way out.

When you look at a scene, you first recognize its general features and identify it as a city street or a suburb or farmland, because of the type of objects it contains. If it's a familiar place, you may recognize specific buildings. But even if you don't, you will still know what it is, because within the scene there are objects, such as lampposts or front lawns or silos, that tell you what the place is meant to do. A lamppost is unlikely to be found in the middle of a field or forest, and a row of corn is unlikely to be found in the middle of a street. When we look at a scene, we not only hunt for such object clues but we also search for narrative, for a story that connects the objects together. If there is something in the scene that doesn't fit, the scene will feel unsettling or magical. When C. S. Lewis, in *The Lion, the Witch and the Wardrobe,* inserts a lamppost in the woods of Narnia, his readers immediately know that this place is not some regular English forest but an extraordinary, magical world.

The brain also perceives nearby things and faraway things in different ways. Stand on a hill overlooking a valley. Distant, medium-range, and close-up objects are recognized in different parts of the brain. The closer ones (house, tree, fountain) are perceived as objects, while the distant features (mountains, skyline) are perceived as a scene. We are constantly scanning the horizon for things that stand out. Such features—the ones that are different—grab our attention and we zoom in on them. Then we zoom back out to view the scene as a whole, scanning all the while. Filmmakers know this. When a filmmaker looks through the camera lens, that lens becomes an extension of the eye—not only the eye of the filmmaker but the eye of each viewer who will later watch the film. A film is visually boring if it is shot from a distance and from only one angle. The camera needs to focus on different parts of the scene—from far to near, to extreme close-up, and then back to far again—to convey depth and realism. This is because our own vision works that way.

Is there something about the structure of a scene that might be intrinsically jarring or relaxing—that could change your mood or affect healing? Indeed, there is a pathway at the base of the brain that leads from the visual cortex to the parahippocampal place area—from the region where signals from the retina are first received to where they are finally constructed into a scene. The nerve cells along this pathway express an increasing density of receptors for endorphins—the brain's own morphine-like molecules. Professor Irving Biederman at the University of Southern California in Los Angeles has found that when people view scenes that are universally preferred—a beautiful vista, a sunset, a grove of trees—the nerve cells in that opiate-rich pathway become active. It is as if when you're looking at a beautiful scene, your own brain gives you a morphine high! Not only that, but as color, depth, and movement are added to the scene, more and more waves of nerve cells become active farther along this opiate-rich gradient.

Could the arrangement of objects in a scene make a difference to the reaction of the viewer, whether consciously or unconsciously? A team of Japanese researchers from the University of Kyoto tackled this question, and used complex mathematics to analyze the structure of an ancient Japanese Zen meditation garden. They published their findings in the journal *Nature* in 2002. The dry-landscape garden at the Ryoanji Temple in Kyoto was laid out during the Muromachi era, which extended from the early fourteenth century to the late sixteenth century. The garden is composed of five irregular clusters of rock, arranged, seemingly haphazardly, on a bare rectangular plot covered with fine gravel raked into patterns. There are few colors or plants, and no flowers, to distract the gaze. The scene was designed to be viewed from the central hall of the temple, which is set oddly askew and slightly to the left of the garden. For centuries, the placement of the rocks was thought to symbolize various things: a tigress crossing the sea with her cubs; the Chinese characters for "heart" or "mind." But no one really knew the meaning of the arrangement, or why the view was so restful.

When the Kyoto researchers analyzed the axes of symmetry between the groups of rock, using a method from image processing called medial-axis transformation, they made a remarkable discovery. The axes formed the shape of a tree whose trunk passed through the central hall of the temple at precisely the spot from which the garden was intended to be viewed. From the main trunk extended "branches," axes that passed between the clusters of rock; the branchings were exactly alike in form, only smaller, as they ramified. When the researchers electronically scrambled the image and scattered the rock clusters randomly, the axes of symmetry were lost. Others have found similar patterns in abstract art.

Such branching, self-similar patterns that occur repeatedly at increasingly smaller scales are found throughout nature, not only in trees but also in waves, snowflakes, seashells, and flowers. They are called *fractals*. The great nineteenth-century Japanese artist Katsushika Hokusai incorporated fractals in his famous woodblock print of crashing waves with Mount Fuji in the distance *(The Great Wave Off Kanagawa)*. Look at this image and you will find the curlicue pattern of waves repeated almost endlessly at smaller and smaller scales. Other fractal structures in nature include mountain ranges, coastlines, the veins in leaves, and the cells in the human body. Nerve cells have a fractal structure, with their ever smaller branches; so too does the circulatory system, with its many self-similar branchings of vessels. Even the human brain is fractal, with its countless replicated folds.

We don't know why repeating patterns are pleasing to the eye, but perhaps their existence in the natural world accounts, in part, for the calming influence of nature views. Such patterns are often found in creative and artistic endeavors. Ary Goldberger, a professor of cardiology at Harvard Medical School and a researcher into heart-rate variability, complexity, and chaos theory, has proposed that fractals are intrinsically satisfying to the human mind. In a paper published in *Molecular Psychiatry* in 1996, he pointed out that Gothic architecture is fractal—with its crenellations, its many self-similar iterations of design, its "porous 'holeyness' or carved-out appearance," its repetition of varied shapes, such as arches and spires, on different scales. Goldberger suggested that when we gaze at fractal structures, whether Gothic cathedrals or Hokusai's waves, our mind responds to the complex, repetitive, increasing-decreasing patterns. Freed from rigid boundaries of scale, the mind can move inward or outward, up or down, at will.

Unlike Zen dry-landscape gardens or Gothic cathedrals, which are largely shades of gray, most of nature is filled with a riot of color. Other kinds of gardens are filled with red roses and orange poppies, blue violets and purple pansies, pink and white impatiens and yellow daffodils, and every possible shade of green. Gardens are also filled with light—dappled light, full sun, and soft, setting sun. Cathedrals have their panoply of color too, concentrated in the intense hues of their stained-glass windows. Why do we feel the need to surround ourselves with light and color, whether in our built environment or in the living world around us? Can light and color affect mood? Can they affect healing? If so, how?

The notion that color can affect mood is not new. Colors on the walls around us, in the clothing we wear, in all the objects we see, as well as the various wavelengths in ambient light—all can influence our emotions.

We perceive color through the cone cells in our retina, which contain pigments that absorb different wavelengths of light. There are three pigments, each of which has the ability to sense a different wavelength: blue, green, or red.

The discovery that different pigments were necessary for color vision came from the recognition that certain people, mostly men, are color blind—that is, they have difficulty identifying colors, and confuse some colors with others. The British king George III, in a letter he wrote to one of his courtiers in 1785, marveled that "the Duke of Marlborough actually cannot tell scarlet from green!" He added that he didn't think this defect ran in the duke's family.

One of the most famous cases of colorblindness was that of the chemist John Dalton, born in England in 1766, who is well known for formulating the atomic theory, which he proposed in 1803 and on which all modern chemistry is based. Atomic weight is still measured in terms of "daltons" or "kilodaltons." But his name is also linked to an inherited form of colorblindness known as *daltonism*. Dalton thought red sealing wax was the same color as a green laurel leaf, and he perceived certain pink geraniums as sky blue. In 1798, he presented a paper to the Manchester Literary and Philosophical Society describing his difficulties seeing colors. He postulated that the vitreous humor in his eyes—the liquid between the lens and retina—was tinted blue, absorbing the longer (red) wavelengths. In his will he instructed that, after his death, his eyes be dissected and the shade of the vitreous humor be examined. His physician, Joseph Ransome, followed this request, sliced one eyeball, and found the vitreous humor to be clear and colorless. He left the second eyeball practically intact. There it sat, desiccating in air, for almost two hundred years, first at Dalton Hall and then in the vaults of the Manchester Literary and Philosophical Society. In the 1990s, researchers from the University of London and from Cambridge University analyzed its DNA. They found that Dalton was missing the gene that codes for one of the photopigments—the one that detects the color green. They published their report in the journal *Science* in February 1995, affirming that Dalton was a *deuteranope*—someone who lacks the middle-wavelength pigment in his retina.

Dalton's brother shared his inability to distinguish certain colors. George III was right to suspect that colorblindness might run in a family. Today we know that the genes for colorblindness are inherited and that the most common ones reside on the X (or female) chromosome. The deficiency usually occurs in males because boys inherit only one X chromosome from their mother, and when an individual has only one copy of the gene and when that copy is defective, only the defective gene will be expressed. Females can be colorblind only if they inherit two copies of the mutated gene, one from their mother and one from their father—and this is a much rarer occurrence.

Each gene codes for a different pigment molecule, made up of two parts. The first is a protein called an *opsin*, which responds to one of the wavelengths of light; the second is a molecule that derives from Vitamin A, the vitamin found in carrots and spinach. When photons (the tiny packets or bursts of light that constitute a lightwave) fall upon their corresponding pigment, the energy sets the pigment molecule vibrating and changes its shape. This triggers a cascade of biochemical events just below the cell's surface, sending an electrical impulse to the parts of the brain that recognize color. When the right wavelength of light hits the pigment that is tuned to match it, the cell starts firing electrical signals. The farther the wavelength is from that perfect match, the slower the firing rate of the cell. So shades of color are translated into electrical signals of various frequencies. The electrical signal then moves up the chain of nerve cells to the visual cortex. As it does so, features are added to the perception. The image is "filled in" with depth, texture, contour, color—all the qualities that enable object recognition.

With just three pigments, we can see all the colors of the rainbow and all the colors in the artist's palette. This ability stems from the two ways the brain blends and compares the signals it receives from each type of pigment cell: it can add or it can subtract. Paints are made up of pigments that absorb certain wavelengths of light and reflect others—the visible colors. When you look at a painting of a green leaf, the green paint is reflecting green wavelengths and absorbing everything else. This is called *color subtraction*. When you mix all the paints together, all the colors are absorbed and you see black. But when you see a colored light, as in a rainbow or on the LCD screen of your computer, you are looking directly at the wavelengths of light. Mix together light of yellow and blue wavelengths and you get green. This is *color addition*. If you mix all the colors in the rainbow, you get white—the blinding bright white of a sunny day. We see the colors separately in a rainbow because each droplet of water in the air is a prism that splits the light into its component wavelengths.

There are many theories as to why a mere three pigments in the color cells of humans (and some primates) can together account for the entire visual spectrum. A clue is embedded in the history of our genes. It turns out that each pigment gene emerged at a different time during evolution. Geneticists know this because genes mutate at a regular rate, so the longer a gene has been around, the more variations in sequencing it contains. Because the time needed for a gene to mutate is fairly standard, scientists can calculate backward from the existing structure to estimate when the gene first appeared.

The photoreceptor pigment gene that emerged first in evolutionary history is the one most sensitive to the spectral distribution of sunlight and to the wavelengths of light reflected from green plants (the yellow-green range). The second to emerge, about 500 million years ago, added to our ability to distinguish many subtle shades of green; it responds to the shorter wavelengths of light (the blue range). The last to emerge, 30–40 million years ago, is the one that responds to the longer wavelengths (the orange-red range). This last gene and the pigment it encodes may have emerged in primates at a time when they began to eat fruit and so had to distinguish bright yellows, oranges, and reds from the background greens of the forest.

If the evolutionary story told within our genes is true, it is not surprising that so much of what the eye is constructed to see falls within the wavelengths of the color green. As a species, humans grew up in forests and fields, in spaces filled with countless shades of green. When a child paints a tree in a single shade of green, the image looks flat. To capture reality, an artist must add many nuances of color—and this is what the eye responds to when we view a forest or field. You can tell the seasons by the shade of green. There is the pale yellow-green of fresh young leaves, the darker green of a mature leaf, the blue-green of spruce needles, the dark green of the underside of a shade tree, the variegated green-and-yellow of a waving field of late-summer prairie grass. You can also tell the time of day by looking at the shade of green of a leafy tree: yellow-green in early morning, when the sun shines through the translucent leaves; shiny, glinting, bright green reflected off the leaves in the noonday sun; shadowed, dark green at dusk, as the sunlight fades.

Only in very recent times have we begun to fill our landscape with other colors, which in urban settings largely displace the green: reflective glass and gunmetal steel, red bricks and gray concrete, black pavement and white sidewalks. Perhaps the color green is the default mode for our brains. It was the background we were weaned on in primordial times, the background that told us we were safe, the background that lulled us to sleep against a darkening sky. Could this be why we find green so relaxing? Could this be why patients with views of trees heal faster than those with views of a brick wall?

Quick recognition of contrasting colors is necessary for survival in the wild, especially in the case of animals that forage for fruit. It is no accident that most fruits contrast starkly with the green foliage around them. Because of their color, fruits are quickly noticed by the animals that eat them and, in the process of digestion and elimination, spread the fruits' seeds. The amazing parsimony of evolution is that this behavior, induced in the animal on the plant's behalf, takes advantage of the skills of the animal's nervous system so that both the eaten and the eater perpetuate their kind.

If you are missing the gene that encodes the green pigment, will you be less likely to feel soothed by the color green? If you are missing the red pigment, will you be less excited by the color red? How do light and color become connected to a mood? Is green naturally soothing and red exciting, or is this response something that we learn? Probably it is a little of both. For many years, operating rooms were painted green, a color that would give the surgeons' eyes a rest from intense gazing at a field of red (the red of the patients' blood and tissues), since green and red are complementary—two colors opposite on the color wheel, with greatest contrast to each other. And green was thought to be a soothing color, since it reflected the hues of nature. Red and yellow were thought to be stimulating colors that promoted alertness. Little systematic research has been done to prove these notions, but the ideas make sense. Much of the information available comes out of marketing and business research. One consistent finding is that shorter-wavelength colors, such as blue and violet, are more appealing to shoppers than longer-wavelength colors like orange and red. As colors move farther to the extremes of wavelength, whether long or short, they become more stimulating, while those in the middle are calming.

A particularly ingenious study was carried out in March 2006, at the *Architectural Digest* Home Design Show in New York City. A consortium including designers, architects, technical staff, a psychologist, a color scientist, and a color lighting expert developed a live-lab color experiment for the show. They set up three identical all-white rooms, eighteen by twenty feet in area and ten feet tall, as cocktail party spaces, each with an identical bar, twelve bar stools, and four computers on pedestals. Several major paint companies were asked to provide the researchers with a list of their most popular shades of red, blue, and yellow. One shade of each color, common to all of the companies, was selected from the list. The outside door panel of each room was painted with one of the colors, and the inside of the room was bathed in colored light to match. Visitors to the design show were free to enter any of the rooms they wished, in any order, and to spend as much time in them as they liked. Observers then documented a range of behaviors on the part of the people who entered the rooms, including food and beverage consumption, choice of room they entered first, ambient sound levels in the rooms, and interactions between occupants. Heart rate was measured with a wristband monitor, and the participants filled out questionnaires on their moods and emotions.

The results of the study seemed to support the general consensus that blue is calming and red and yellow are stimulating. Twice as many people entered the yellow room compared to the blue room. While people reported feeling more hungry and thirsty in the red room, food and beverage consumption was twice as high in the yellow room. People in the blue room reported feeling calm, or used the word "calm," significantly more often than people in the yellow and red rooms. People also clustered differently in the three rooms. In the blue room, they spent more time standing around the perimeter, while in the yellow and red rooms they spent more time clustered in the middle. People in the yellow room were the most animated; they moved around more, and spent more time talking and laughing loudly in small groups, than those in the other rooms. They described their moods as "active," "playful," "energetic." The physiological measure, heart rate, did not change. While this study has many strengths, especially its comparison of objective measures of responses to identical spaces of different color, most likely it was measuring the effects of exposure to light of different wavelengths, rather than exposure to color on the walls. So while it may not show how different room colors might affect behavior and mood, it does suggest that different wavelengths of light have these effects. It would be interesting to repeat the experiment using various wall colors instead of colored lights.

If colors evoke emotions, the association between the two is probably something we have learned. A color can get attached to a mood when cone cells send signals to the visual centers in the brain that recognize the color, and along the way some electrical impulses travel to the brain's emotional centers. The excitement and craving we feel when looking at an image of a luscious fruit arises from the same parts of the brain that control desire of any sort. These are the parts of the brain that become active when a chocoholic craves chocolate, when a smoker craves cigarettes, when a drinker craves alcohol, or when a drug addict craves heroin. They are among the brain's reward pathways, and they also become active when we crave sex. The chemical that is released from nerve cells in these parts of the brain is called *dopamine*.

Activity in the brain's reward pathways can get attached to colors through a form of learning called *classical conditioning*. The Russian scientist and physician Ivan Pavlov first described this type of learning in the 1890s; he won the Nobel Prize in Physiology in 1904 for this discovery. Conditioning will be familiar to anyone who has ever owned a pet. It explains why dogs and cats associate the sound of a can opener with dinner. Pavlov's method is the basis of all behavioral training. Show a dog a steak and it salivates. Ring a bell and nothing happens. Ring a bell at the same moment you present the steak, and the dog will salivate. Repeat this pairing a few times. Then merely ring the bell, and the dog will salivate. The dog has learned to associate the sound of the bell with the tasty steak. This happens in humans too, more often than we realize. It is this form of conditioning that could link a color to a certain mood.

Pavlov's experiments proved that a learned neutral stimulus, like the sound of a bell, could be paired with a physiological response, such as salivation and hunger. Scientists needed more than a century to learn how this circuit works in human appetite. It turns out that hormones released from the stomach play a crucial role in amplifying and changing brain pathways involved in this response.

When you look at a picture of an apple, the reward parts of the brain become active only if you are hungry. If you have just eaten a satisfying meal and are shown the picture, those desire parts of your brain remain silent. When your stomach fills with food, nerves in the wall of the stomach tell your brain that the stomach muscles are stretched, and you feel sated. As food is broken down, the body releases many chemicals and hormones that signal your brain to stop eating—substances like sugars, insulin, and the hormones ghrelin and leptin. *Ghrelin* increases appetite when you are hungry. *Leptin,* produced by cells in the stomach after you have eaten, travels through the bloodstream to the hypothalamus and other parts of the brain that control appetite, and quenches your desire to eat. If a hungry person is given an injection of leptin while looking at a picture of a ripe

juicy fruit, the desire parts of the brain, which were active a moment before, become quiet.

This feature of the way the things we see are connected to
powerful emotional responses has been exploited by marketers
around the world. Everyone knows the old adage, "Never go to
the grocery store when you're hungry"—you'll buy much more
food than you intended. This is because the pictures of food on
the containers are designed to entice you to buy, and they tempt
you much more when you are hungry. It took a long while for
the military to apply this principle to the food packages that it
distributed to the troops in the field. For many years MREs
(Meals Ready to Eat) came in dull, khaki-green packages. A sol-
dier under stress has little appetite to begin with, and troops receiving these rations had a tendency to throw away most of the
food. When the U.S. Army's food scientists developed attractive
packages like the ones on grocery store shelves, the soldiers
showed greater interest in their food and improved their nutritional intake. Marketers take advantage of other features of visual perception, such as size and position. Walk into a department store and you are surrounded by objects vying for your
attention. The ones you'll notice are the ones placed directly in
your field of vision. They are often large, bright, glittery, or
high-contrast.

Of course, it is not just color but also the shape and associations of an image which are stimulating. When you are hungry,
a picture of a red apple will excite your brain, but one of a
red brick will not. This is because you have learned to associate
the image of a red apple with something tasty and sweet. Researchers have taken advantage of this principle to train people
to associate the color of a drinking glass with its contents, either
alcohol or sweetened water. Once individuals learn the association, they react to a glass of a certain color as if they are drinking
an alcoholic beverage (mild craving, sweaty skin, attention fo-

cused on the glass), even if they're actually drinking mere sweetened water.

What if you were unable to see the color red? Would you be less likely to be tempted by that apple or that beverage? Ask colorblind individuals this question, and they will emphatically answer no. They can still recognize an apple, and know that it would taste good. They can still learn to associate a colored glass with an alcoholic beverage. Just think of the times you have watched a black-and-white television show. You quickly forget that it's black-and-white, and your mind matches the shades of gray to colors you would expect to see. People who are born missing one of their photopigments are just as tempted by a juicy red apple as those whose color vision is intact. The color they see may be different from the one the rest of us see, but they will still have learned to associate it with an emotional response.

If it is difficult to pin down whether and how various hues might affect mood, it is much easier to determine how mood could respond to different wavelengths, intensities, and rhythms of light. For centuries, northern Europeans have been vacationing in Italy, Greece, and Spain to escape the winter darkness of their own countries. The sunlight draws them there, the same brightness that so many painters have captured in their works—Tintoretto, Bellini, Titian, Leonardo da Vinci. Indeed, the Mediterranean countries are virtually synonymous with sunlight. Every year, "snowbirds" from across the Northern Hemisphere head south to shorten their winters and lift their mood.

Northern artists like Rembrandt were famous for their paintings filled with rich, shadowy tints, with figures highlighted by a single shaft of light or a flickering fire. Northern countries are afflicted with gloom, not only in the weather but also in mood. There is a high rate of depression and suicide in Scandinavian countries, some say because of the long winters and Arctic nights. There is a form of depression called *seasonal affective disorder* (SAD) which is brought on by lack of sunlight or by prolonged exposure to artificial light or darkness. People with SAD feel fatigued, depressed, and listless. Their brain's stress hormones are sluggish and tuned too low. This might sound like a good thing, but in fact you need your stress hormones to give you energy and keep you alert. Exposure to bright sunlight, or to lights that have the same intensity and wavelength spectrum as sunlight, can be used to treat patients with this form of depression, preventing slumps in mood, restoring energy, and bringing stress hormones back to normal.

The hormones and nerve chemicals released from various centers in the brain ebb and flow naturally, in sync with the ebb and flow of light and dark, just as the tides rise and fall with the time of day and the sun and moon. These rhythms of our body are in tune with the rhythms of the sun. As daylight ebbs, so too do many hormones. Just before dawn, these hormones start flowing again; they peak in the early morning, gradually decline throughout the day, and bottom out in the evening. They're the reason you need a cup of coffee at the end of the afternoon. This natural cycling is called *circadian rhythm,* a term derived from the Latin for "about a day."

If your internal clock is out of adjustment, you'll wake up in the middle of the night. Think of what happens when you fly from New York to Honolulu. For the first few days you get sleepy at 4:00 in the afternoon and wake up at 2:00 in the morning, because your hormonal bursts are still set on New York time. It takes a few days for your brain to catch up and start working on the rhythm of the new cycles. You can speed this process by forcing yourself to stay awake and walking about in the bright sun. The hormone *melatonin* can also help to reset your clock.

Melatonin is a tiny molecule made from the amino acid

tryptophan. It pulses through the bloodstream at night and helps you sleep, increasing in the early evening, peaking in the hours from midnight to 4:00 A.M., then gradually falling to its lowest levels just before dawn. In "night owls," people who are active at night, this cycle occurs later; in "morning larks," who function well in the morning, the peak comes earlier in the evening. In teenagers, the pattern shifts even later in the night, so they have trouble getting up much before noon.

Melatonin is released from cells in the pineal gland, one of the clock centers in your brain. The pineal is not really brain tissue; it's a gland buried in the center of the brain, between the two hemispheres. Long ago, people thought it was a vestige of a third eye sported by some primordial ancestor, such as a Cyclops, because although it lies deep within the skull, it responds to rhythms of light. When you fly from New York to Honolulu, your pineal gland keeps pumping out melatonin at the same rhythm and times that it followed when you were in New York, until gradually it has a chance to reset. It's like time travel in reverse: your body has traveled to Honolulu, but your pineal gland is still in New York.

The brain's clock center and stress center are likewise reset in clinical depression. In SAD they are set too low, and the rhythm flattens. In the more common form of depression called *melancholic depression,* they are set too high and kick in too early in the night. If you're clinically depressed, you wake up in the middle of the night for no apparent reason, feeling wide awake. Later, during the day, you feel a slump and become drowsy at times when you should be attending to work or family or chores. When you're awake in the wee hours, you may note the time on your bedside clock, then look out the window and see that it's still dark outside. Loops of worry start inside your head—worry about yourself and all the things you didn't do and should have done, and all the things you've done but shouldn't have. You may feel your heart start beating fast, and when you get up to go to the bathroom, you start to pace—too full of energy to go back to sleep. It's your stress hormones that are making you feel this way, for they as well, driven by the brain's circadian clock, start pumping out too early in the night.

Some of this cycling is linked to light-sensitive proteins in the eye, similar to the ones that register color. These proteins are found in the nerve cells of the retina, two or three layers beneath the rods and cones. They respond to light much more slowly and evenly than do the ones that register color, and they are best at detecting light intensity rather than color. These cells may be the ones that link the circadian clock to the light cycles of the day. There are also direct nerve connections between these cells in the eye and the parts of the brain that regulate circadian rhythms. Some nerve cells from the retina send their long fibers to the brain's stress center, and also to the brain's main clock center. Other nerve fibers lead from there to areas in the brain stem that regulate the rhythms of the heart.

Besides lifting moods and changing stress hormones, full-spectrum sunlight can also change the heart rhythm in people with SAD—not the heart rate, but rather the time intervals between beats. These intervals reflect the activation state of the nerves that speed and slow the heart—the adrenalin-like nerves of the sympathetic nervous system and the vagus nerve. Certain wavelengths of light can also shift heart rhythms in people without depression. In one study, researchers exposed healthy participants to ten minutes of light of red, green, or blue wavelengths and then measured heart-rate variability. They found that the red and green wavelengths had a stimulating effect and that the blue ones were calming. This matched subjective reports from the participants, who found the blue light relaxing and the red and green energizing. This finding is surprisingly similar to the marketing studies which showed that shoppers prefer blue and violet to red and yellow.

Just as sunlight can boost moods and physiological responses, a dearth of sunlight can lower them. Prolonged exposure to fluorescent lighting in the absence of natural light, a common situation in office spaces, can dampen moods in most people, even those without clinical SAD. This is especially so in late fall and in winter, when, because of daylight savings time, many people leave for work before dawn, spend all day in artificial lighting, and return home after dark. Researcher Michael Terman, at Columbia University, found a higher incidence of depression and mood disorders not only among people in northern latitudes, but also among people living at the far western edge of their time zone, where the sun rises an hour later than at the eastern end. It seems that the resetting of our pineal clock depends upon the timing of the dawn and on our exposure to bright sunlight when we awake, rather than on the timing of the setting of the sun.

Light has been proven to affect not only the mood of office workers and shoppers, but also the length of hospital stay in patients with depression, even if the form of depression was not seasonal affective disorder. Researchers conducted two studies of depressed patients on hospital wards in which half of the rooms were bright and sunny and the other half had low light. They reported significantly shortened hospital stays for the patients who had been in the sunny rooms. The locations of the studies could not have been farther apart: one was carried out in 1996 in Edmonton, Canada, where in winter the temperature can dip to minus 25 degrees Centigrade and light intensities are amplified over a four-month period by reflection from the snow. The other was carried out in 2001 in Milan, Italy, where morning sun in early summer can produce light intensities of more than 15,000 lux (compared to 2,500–5,000 lux for artificial light). By chance, in the Italian study, the rooms on one side of the ward faced east and were lit by the morning sun, while the rooms on the other side of the ward faced west and received direct light only from the setting sun, in the range of 150–3,000 lux. In the Canadian study, all of the rooms had large windows, but, much as in Roger Ulrich's 1984 study, half of the rooms faced a glass-roofed courtyard and the other half had an outdoor view. In the Italian study, patients who suffered from bipolar depression and who had been housed in east-facing rooms were discharged more than three and a half days sooner than bipolar patients who had been in west-facing rooms. This was not the case for patients with unipolar depression, in whom no effect of sunlight was observed. In Alberta, where patients with all forms of depression were included, the patients who had stayed in brighter rooms left the hospital more than two and a half days sooner than depressed patients who had been in rooms with low light.

Working a night shift can have deleterious effects on health. So too can spending a large proportion of time changing time zones, as pilots and flight attendants do. In 2005, Richard Stevens at the University of Connecticut found that women who spent their working lives on night shift had a 30–80 percent greater chance of developing breast cancer than those who worked regular hours. In September 2006, Stevens and a team of scientists convened by the National Institute of Environmental Health Sciences concluded that full-spectrum lighting can be used to treat many syndromes and mood disorders related to insufficient or disrupted exposure to sunlight. Their work inspired the International Agency for Research on Cancer, a committee of the World Health Organization, to study the topic. The agency found strong evidence that shift work is linked to cancer, though no one knows the reasons for this association or whether light therapy could be beneficial in such situations.

Besides changing our moods and our behavior, light can also affect our immune systems. In so doing, it can change the way we heal. The heliotherapy of the early twentieth century did help healing, but not of tuberculosis, as its proponents thought. When light touches us, it triggers chemical reactions in the body's cells at the spot where it falls, just as it triggers chemical reactions in the photoreceptors in the eye. We all recognize the effect of too much sunlight on the skin: a sunburn. When too much light falls on us—bright noonday tropical sunlight, for example—the packets of light penetrate molecules of DNA in skin cells, and break them apart. This cooking process triggers inflammation. The immune system recognizes the bits and pieces of DNA as foreign, as something not our own, and sends inflammatory cells to clean them up. Blood vessels dilate, and the skin at the site becomes engorged and red and tender. White blood cells stream in and proceed to clear the damaged tissue. If enough damage has been done, serum oozes out from blood vessels and blisters appear. Eventually, with repeated DNA damage and repair, errors occur in the genetic code, and the result is skin cancer.

While too much light is harmful, a little sunlight on the skin is a good thing. If there is enough energy to set some molecules vibrating but not enough to burn, it can help us heal. Vitamin D is one of the molecules that is activated by light falling on the skin—but only by shorter wavelengths, those in the ultraviolet range. Vitamin D is essential for getting calcium into bones. It also strengthens the immune system, especially the macrophages, which chew up debris during inflammation. When fed Vitamin D, these cells spew out immune molecules that summon other immune cells, and thus speed healing.

So here is a dilemma: How can we avoid too much short-wavelength exposure (and possible skin cancer), while getting enough sunlight to activate the Vitamin D we need for growth and healing? This is a particular problem in children, who can suffer severe defects for lack of Vitamin D: weak bones, short stature, and abnormal bone growth, especially in the legs. The illness resulting from Vitamin D deficiency, called *rickets,* was recognized in the seventeenth century, long before its cause was finally discovered, in the early twentieth century. It was largely eradicated by adding Vitamin D to milk and other foods.

Recently, there has been an alarming increase in Vitamin D deficiency in many countries. Children are developing rickets; adult women show symptoms of fatigue and weakness, joint and muscle aches, and weak bones—symptoms that overlap with those of chronic-fatigue syndrome and fibromyalgia, and can include symptoms of depression. The Mayo Clinic researchers who in 2003 reported these findings in women in the United States suggested that the rise in such illnesses may be due to de-creased consumption of milk and dairy products and, as an edi-torial in the same journal suggested, overuse of sunblock and avoidance of sunlight from fear of cancer. All of this underscores the importance of balance: while too much sun can lead to DNA damage and too little can cause vitamin deficiencies, a certain amount is necessary for good health.

Our brains and bodies contain circuitry which allows the light around us to change our moods, the rhythms of our stress re-sponse, and the way our immune cells fight infection. Exposure to light and to certain visual scenes may in part explain how the view through a hospital window could speed healing. But what about sounds? Birds chirping, rain pattering on the window ledge, foliage rustling in the breeze? Could these, too, help us heal?

3

SOUND AND SILENCE

Silence. Is it emptiness? Is it nothing? When you listen to the silence around you in a quiet place, what you really hear are the tiny sounds that are usually drowned out by background noise: dry leaves blowing across the pavement, the crunch of pebbles beneath your feet, the call of a bird, the skitter of a tiny creature on the path, the wind in the trees. If you close your eyes, you can tell the seasons or the time of day. You can tell if it's spring or fall from the way the wind rustles through the trees. In fall, the leaves sound crisp; in spring, they are silky soft and the breeze flowing through them is almost inaudible. On a summer night the crickets' rhythmic chirping seems to come from all around, and rises and falls like waves upon the air. At dawn the birds take over—a cacophony of song you never hear in the heat of midday. In quiet places, we hear the life around us and come into closer contact with our world. We are in touch with nature, in tune with our thoughts, and aware of forces greater than ourselves. As Henry David Thoreau said in *Walden* (1854), the book he wrote while living alone in the forest: "I wish to hear the silence of the night, for the silence is something positive and to be heard. . . . The silence rings. It is musical and thrills me."

But when you are sick in bed in a hospital room, you do not hear these things. You certainly do not hear silence. At precisely the moment you are craving peace and quiet, you hear all sorts of noises—loud noises. The sound in intensive-care units can range from forty-five to ninety-eight decibels: the clatter and whir of machinery, the click of heels on hard-tiled floors, tele-phones ringing, human voices reverberating off walls and ceil-ings and metallic countertops. All through the night, you hear doctors and nurses going about their daily rounds, the chatter of visitors in the hallways, the moaning of other patients in pain. None of these are comforting sounds. None of them remind you of home and health.

Our perception of sounds begins in the sensory organ de-signed specifically for this purpose: the ear—an incredibly deli-cate and complex instrument that detects movements of air molecules and the differences in frequency and pitch that the movements create. When a pulse of sound reaches the ears, it gets funneled into the auditory canal by the *pinnae,* the fleshy protuberances that every schoolchild draws as semicircles stick-ing out on either side of the head. In humans this part of the ear is less agile than in dogs or cats or bats, which can quickly turn their pinnae toward a sound to capture it. The next thing the waves of air hit is the *tympanum,* a tightly stretched membrane that's located at the end of the external auditory canal and that vibrates like a drum. Hence its name: eardrum. The air distur-bances hit your eardrums and make them vibrate at the same fre-quency as the sound, much the way stereo speakers vibrate with music. But instead of being connected to a speaker, the eardrum is connected to three tiny, loosely hinged bones inside the next chamber, the middle ear. Each bone is delicate and exquisitely shaped. One looks like a hammer and is called by its Latin name, *malleus.* The next, the *incus,* looks like an anvil. And the third, the *stapes,* looks like a stirrup. When the eardrum vibrates, these bones vibrate in tune with its movement and with the move-ment of the air.

In the last chamber, the inner ear, the sound waves reach a carpet of cells. These cells have very fine filaments that wave above the carpet like blades of grass. They are called *hair cells,* and this organ, the real organ of hearing, is called the *basilar membrane of the cochlea* because it is a flat, ribbon-like structure that winds around in a spiral, like a snail shell (*kochlias* in Greek). Each filament is a different thickness and thus vibrates best at a different frequency, just as each string on a guitar vibrates at a different frequency according to its thickness. In the final step, the vibrating hairs trigger electrical impulses in the fibers of the auditory nerve cells on which they sit. The rate of firing corresponds to the frequency of the hairs' vibrations. And so, through this chain of tiny musical instruments, from eardrum through middle ear to inner ear, air movements are translated into electrical signals that travel along nerve pathways throughout the brain.

As the electrical signals are handed off from one nerve cell to the next, they divide into *where* streams (nerve cells that tell you where a sound is coming from) and *what* streams (nerve cells that tell you what the sound is). Bats are particularly good at detecting where a sound is coming from, while primates, including humans, are better at detecting what a sound is. We can locate sounds—and in turn use them to locate ourselves in space—because we hear in stereo. A sound will arrive at one ear just a few thousandths of a second sooner than it arrives at the other ear. The auditory centers in our brains are able to detect this slight discrepancy and employ it to determine where a sound is coming from. A moving sound also gets louder as it approaches us and softer as it draws away from us. Think of an ambulance on a city street—you know how far away it is by the loudness of the siren.

The part of the brain where sounds are interpreted is called the *auditory cortex*. It lies in a region known as the *temporal lobe*. As its name suggests, this is the area behind the temples, toward the middle of your head, just under the skullbone behind your ears. Just as visual signals from the retina maintain their spatial organization all the way to the brain, so the keyboard-like layout of the hair cells in the cochlea, extending from low pitch to high, is maintained through these auditory switching stations all the way to the auditory cortex, which contains a pitch keyboard much like that in the cochlea. There tones are laid out from low to high frequency, in an arrangement called a *tonotopic map*.

Marc Raichle, a neurologist at Washington University in St. Louis and also an accomplished pianist, was among the first researchers to demonstrate this layout. In the late 1970s and early 1980s, he was one of a small group of pioneers who used PET scans to study brain function and blood flow. In this type of brain imaging, high-energy radioactive compounds are injected into the bloodstream and decompose within minutes. A scanner that detects radioactivity constructs an instantaneous picture of blood flow in regions where nerve cells are active. When Raichle exposed research participants to a series of pure tones much like a piano scale, he was amazed: areas of blood flow became active in an arrangement that looked just like a piano keyboard. This map-like representation of blood flow corresponded to the regions of the brain where nerve cells were firing in an orderly fashion according to pitch. He had achieved a first glimpse of blood flow to the tonotopic map!

Early in the process, before a sound signal reaches the auditory cortex but after it leaves the hair cells, the streams of nerve cells divide, some branching toward the speech areas in the brain and others toward areas that are specialized for detection of musical features. *Feature extraction* is a very important part of how we perceive sound, just as it is essential to how we see. The speech areas deconstruct sounds into the individual units that constitute spoken language—the phonemes that make up words—while the music areas detect those elements of sound that make up music, including pitch, timbre, contour, and rhythm. Some streams take a shortcut to the part of the brain that measures timing. Others flow to the various emotion centers in the brain. And thus sounds, particularly music, can trigger many different emotional responses.

In the rolling hills just north of Boston, a small oval pond lies hidden in the woods. Since the late nineteenth century, the locals have used this swimming hole to escape the heat of summer. The water is surprisingly warm. But as you push your inner tube toward the middle of the lake to escape the squishy, weedy bottom near the shore, fingers of cold water brush against you. These come from the spring that bubbles up to feed the pond.

The little pond is drained at the south end by a nameless brook that runs through wetlands filled in summer with purple loosestrife, skunk cabbage, delicate jewelweed, and St. John's Wort. The brook flows south and empties into a small river called the Spicket. This feeds into the Merrimack, which, after meandering through salty sand flats, joins the Atlantic Ocean northeast of Boston. The Merrimack was, and still is, a main commercial transport route through central New England.

It was because of rivers like the Merrimack and their tributaries that in the mid-1800s German, Irish, and French Canadian settlers came to this area at the height of the Industrial Revolution. Here they built mills to weave cloth made of cotton, wool, and linen. The falls along the streams and rivers provided the power to turn the water wheels that moved the shuttles of the looms. The huge redbrick buildings still dominate the small cities scattered through these hills—Manchester, Lowell, Lawrence, Methuen, Haverhill.

If you follow the no-name brook to the Spicket and then trace the river south, you come to a spot where it drops suddenly by about forty feet. These falls mark the center of the town of Methuen. An old mill once stood at this site, now a parking lot. On one side of the parking lot stands an imposing redbrick building. It could be a church or maybe the Town Hall, but in fact it is neither. Built in 1909 for an interior designer, railroad magnate, and real estate developer named Edward Searles, the building was constructed with one sole purpose: to house an organ.

Walk up the steps, then through an unimposing entrance foyer, and you find yourself in the back of a sunny auditorium, two stories high, dominated at the north end by an enormous organ made of American black walnut, reaching to the dome. So amazing is this sight that you stop and stare. The wooden case, which supports the thirty-foot-tall pipes arranged in a graceful arc, is richly carved with figures evoking Michelangelo. Two Atlas-like torsos strain to support the tallest pipes to the left and right of the keyboard. A pair of famous composers support the lesser pipes on either side of the stage. Marching toward each side of the stage are stalwart Valkyries with long Teutonic braids and stern faces. And above the center of the stage, a bust of J. S. Bach surveys all in silence.

If you happen to wander into the hall during rehearsal for the July Fourth celebration, you might see the choir practicing under the direction of the church's pastor. He moves quickly back and forth, from conducting the choir to sitting at the organ bench. Hands and feet poised, he gives one last nod to the choir, then drops his hands to the tiered keyboard and lunges forward, simultaneously pressing keys and pedals. Abruptly the hall fills with a great reverberating sound. You are engulfed by the vibrations, which seem to rise up through the floor. You stand motionless and allow them to move up your spine and carry you away. Until Edward Searles died, he was the only person privileged to hear this sound. He had bought the organ and built the hall in memory of his dead wife, who loved music. When Searles sat alone, sunk in reverie, bathed in the sounds of this enormous organ, he was able to reexperience the emotions he had felt when his wife had lived, as well as the profound grief he felt after her death.

How is music able to evoke emotions and memories? And what is it about the first reverberating chords of the organ that stirs the listener so deeply? Where is the source of that awe and surprise, that shivery feeling you get when you hear the organ's first blast?

"Goose bumps. Goose bumps. Goose bumps." These were Daniel Levitin's response when he worked with the musician Carlos Santana, the response that made him leave his career as a successful California recording engineer to study neuroscience. Levitin recalled the exact moment when, preparing to tinker with the sound equipment as Santana played, he felt those goose bumps and asked himself: What was it about the music that had such an effect on him? What was happening in his brain?

Just as with vision, hearing works best when there is contrast. And contrast entails the element of surprise—the jolt we experience when, say, we emerge from a low cramped space into a large open one, or when a quiet hall fills suddenly with sound. It is the astonishment we feel when we are lulled by the warm New England countryside and then abruptly encounter an enormous organ. Our response is both physical and emotional as we're struck by this juxtaposition of low and dark with towering light, of quiet stillness with reverberating sound, of bucolic fields with thundering organ. First you feel a shiver in your spine, and maybe a tingling in your fingers. Then you catch your breath. You inspire and are inspired.

It is the contrast between silence and sound that produces this effect. Had the organ struck its chords in the middle of rush-hour traffic in Manhattan, they would have been barely perceptible. In fact, this is a problem that New York City authorities have struggled with as sound pollution has increased—how to make the sirens of emergency vehicles noticeable above the din. Sirens not only need to be louder but also need a changing *pattern* of sound, in order to be heard.

The reason for this is that, at all levels in the nervous system—a single nerve cell, groups of cells, entire brain regions—what is most detectable is difference. Nerve cells respond better to a sudden change than they do to repeated stimuli of the same kind or intensity. This is true for all our senses.

The difference between the firing rate of a nerve responding to a sound, and the nerve's background firing rate, is called the *signal-to-noise ratio*. In this case, "noise" refers to the low-level chatter of nerve cells' electrical activity, which goes on all the time. The greater the difference between the specific sound signal and the background activity, the more distinctly the sound is heard. Loud sounds, which cause nerve cells to fire at a higher rate, have the greatest signal-to-noise ratio and are more clearly audible than soft sounds. But soft sounds heard in a very quiet environment can have a signal-to-noise ratio that is equally pronounced, and thus they can be heard quite clearly.

Sudden change—a noise, a puff of air—prompts a reaction in all animals called the *startle response*—a reflex similar to the knee jerk that is triggered when the doctor taps your knee with a rubber hammer. You are sitting in your chair, hard at work at your computer, and the office prankster sneaks up behind you and claps his hands loudly. You jump—practically leap out of your seat. If you were to place a digital scale on your seat cushion, you would find that the reflex increases with the intensity of the sound: the louder the sound, the higher you jump and the harder you land. In fact, this is a standard way to test the startle response in animals: a scale is embedded in the floor of the animal's cage. In humans, the intensity of this reflex can be measured by gluing small electrodes on top of the eyelids. Each time you jump, you also blink your eyes, and the intensity of the blink correlates with the degree of startle.

Why would researchers go to such lengths to measure the startle reflex in animals and people? The reason is that this simple reflex is wired by nerve cells in a circuit that runs from the ear through a switching station in the brain stem directly to the brain's fear center, the *amygdala*. Measuring this reflex gives an indication of the intensity of the fear response and is routinely used to test the efficacy of anti-anxiety drugs to block it.

Startle is a very primitive and life-saving reflex, because whenever there is sudden change in the environment, an animal must focus its attention on the scene and must be ready to defend itself or run. The parts of the brain that form this circuit are the same parts that control our attention and prepare our body to flee during the stress response. If a frightening event has been experienced before, the brain's stress center, the *hypothalamus,* instantly gets connected to the circuit and amplifies the startle response. This, too, is life-saving. When you find yourself in a situation that resembles one in which you experienced danger before, your brain's stress center is already wired to recall the setting instantly and place you on alert.

Sometimes we actually seek that feeling of startle and hint of fear, because these are the ingredients of awe, and awe can be thrilling—just frightening enough to excite but not so much as to terrify. Repeated exposure to startling events, though, can cause us to lose the buzz, for the brain is wired to settle into a state of calm when the continual contrasts become monotonous. When we are exposed to many loud noises of the same tone and intensity, the startle response and the nerve-cell firing rates in the brain regions that register sound gradually respond less and less, until they, and we, no longer notice. This is called *habituation*.

It is possible to measure a single nerve cell's electrical response by touching the cell with an electrode made from a very fine glass tube drawn out like angel-hair taffy in a flame. Such electrodes can record the nerve cell's firing in response to any disturbance; the activity shows up as machine-gun-like blips on an oscilloscope. But with monotonous, repeated perturbations, the firing rate diminishes and eventually dies down. Once the cell has habituated, it will not fire up again unless a new stimulus appears, or unless there's a change in the tone or pitch or pattern of the sound.

This is why we can block out monotonous repeated sounds, and why the white noise of a machine such as an air-conditioner can be relaxing. Imagine you're lying in bed at night, tossing and turning because you can't switch off your racing thoughts. A storm begins—no thunder and lightening, just rain hard enough to make itself heard on the roof and windowpanes. You are cozy and warm under a down comforter. You focus on the sound of the rain and soon are fast asleep. Or maybe it's the pounding of waves upon a beach that lulls you to sleep, or the babble of a flowing brook. These sounds all have the same effect. The word "lull," which means a brief interval of calm but can also imply boredom, is the root of "lullaby"—a song that calms an infant and makes it sleepy. Some mothers even report that the sound of a vacuum cleaner helps their babies get to sleep.

The ability of the brain to become habituated to sound has spawned a whole Web industry of downloadable nature sounds called *pink noise,* which can be stored on your iPod or MP3 player in case you need help falling asleep. These recordings are also used to treat people with a form of hearing impairment called *tinnitus,* in which damage to the auditory nerve causes annoying and disturbing sounds in the sufferer's ear. Listening to pink noise can override the shrill notes of tinnitus and give the patient some relief, until the brain finally habituates to the tinnitus itself and treats it like any other background noise.

In sum, the brain is wired to react to sudden change with a burst of electrical activity, which, when flashing through the brain's fear and stress centers, makes us shiver, feel fear, and want to run away. This contrast increases our awareness of the world around us. When all is calm, like the surface of a lake at dusk or a sky without clouds, one barely notices the air. But with a sudden breeze that moves the clouds and churns the surface of the water into waves, we suddenly become aware of air's existence. It is the same with sudden sound that startles us out of inattention to hear the background music. But if all music did was to instill fear or, through habituation, to induce boredom, how could we humans be so addicted to music? How could it excite us?

People have always known that music can alter moods. From the moment musical instruments were first invented, music was used to calm or to terrify. The ancient Greeks, in their temples to the god of healing, Asclepius, used music to help heal the sick. Aristotle and Plato wrote about music's healing power. Music was used for millennia to strengthen the resolve of troops heading into battle. The fife and drum, the bagpipe, the trumpet inspired the attackers and daunted the enemy. Ritual dances accompanied by throbbing music can send people into a sexual frenzy. We know all this from generations of art and culture, but only recently have scientists developed technologies that could be used to understand how emotion and music are connected, and to prove that music can affect moods.

When Daniel Levitin decided to change careers and seek answers to such age-old questions, he first had to trace the brain's pathways for receiving sounds and combining them into a recognizable piece of music. Then he had to trace the pathways by which sounds arrive at the brain's emotion centers. A graduate of the Berklee College of Music, a rock musician who became a record producer and then a neuroscientist, Levitin is now a professor at McGill University.

After dropping out of college in the 1970s, Levitin joined a band that became popular in the San Francisco Bay area, recording several albums. He spent much of his time between takes in the control room with the sound engineer, learning the elements of the trade. When the band broke up, he went on to produce albums by other musicians such as Stevie Wonder, Carlos Santana, and Steely Dan and to consult on Hollywood movie scores.

Levitin was fascinated by the question of why some songs move us and others don't, and how great musicians differ from the rest of us when listening to or making music. He sat in on psychology classes taught by the Stanford neuropsychologist Karl Pribram. Eventually he went back to school and earned a Ph.D. in cognitive psychology from the University of Oregon. He chose to focus directly on the brain, using *functional magnetic resonance imaging* (fMRI), to capture images of brain function as people were listening to music.

Like magnetic resonance imaging, which is used to view anatomical structures in the brain and body for the purpose of diagnosing disease, fMRI relies on the fact that molecules can be made to spin when in a very powerful magnetic field. This kind of imaging not only shows anatomical structures, but also shows whether those structures are active and how active they are. The information is translated into various intensities or shades of color on an image that the radiologist can see.

Unlike PET scans, fMRI does not require that a radioactive tracer be injected into the blood. It relies on the blood's constituent hemoglobin, which in turn contains iron that is slightly magnetic. The body part that is being scanned is exposed to the field of a huge and powerful magnet, which makes the iron atoms spin. The fMRI machine's computer tracks the resulting changes in the magnetic fields of red blood cells as they flow through vessels. When an area lights up on an fMRI scan, this means that more blood is flowing through it—that more nerve cells have become active and are using energy supplied by the blood. As Levitin points out in his book *This Is Your Brain on Music*, ironically the method was developed by the British music company EMI using profits from the sale of their Beatles recordings.

Using this technique, Levitin was able to identify the areas of the brain that become active when a person is listening to music, especially the emotion areas. He was intrigued by how the brain, after it perceives individual features of a sound—pitch, amplitude, direction, timbre, rhythm—puts them all together to create a perception of music. He also wanted to know how a sound can trigger an emotional response.

It turns out that there is no single area devoted to music. The brain is a parallel processor, constantly receiving signals from the ears, analyzing them, and then reconstructing and revising what it perceives. This is similar to the way all the other senses operate. Our perception of the auditory landscape is ever-changing, determined both by the sounds we are exposed to and by our internal state.

In the 1990s, McGill researchers Ann Blood and Robert Zatorre found, using PET scans, that when a person listens to exciting music, several brain regions involved in emotion become active, including the amygdala (the fear center) and the *ventral striatum* (the reward center). These regions constitute the *limbic system* and are among the most primitive circuits in the brain, guiding positive emotions, such as sexual desire and feelings of reward, as well as uncontrollable desires, such as addiction.

Levitin was particularly interested in the *nucleus accumbens,* which lies within one of the main reward regions in the brain. It was not visible in Blood's studies, since PET scanning is unable to detect such a tiny region. But fMRI can do this. So Levitin performed a study in which he exposed people to exciting music and made fMRI scans to see which brain regions became active. As he predicted, the first area to light up was the auditory cortex—the *what* area, which extracts features of sounds. Lighting up next were areas in the front of the brain involved in thought and in deciphering structure. The last to become active were the emotion centers, those involved in arousal and pleasure, including the nucleus accumbens. These are all areas where *dopamine,* the nerve chemical of desire, and the body's natural opioids, the *endorphins,* are released. So it seems that music turns your brain on, both electrically and chemically, and, like any reward, has the capacity to produce feelings of intense desire. When Levitin published his landmark paper, one news outlet announced that he had found the brain's center for "sex, drugs, and rock and roll."

Other nerve chemicals are also involved in our emotional responses to sound. *Serotonin,* which drops to low levels when an individual is depressed, and the adrenalin-like chemical *norepinephrine,* which increases during stress, are not in themselves involved in sound perception, but can profoundly affect the brain's ability to detect features of sound. They also influence vision. In the presence of serotonin, nerve cells tuned to a fuzzy, wide range of frequencies become focused on a narrower range. The signal sharpens and our perception becomes clearer.

Levitin found that the cerebellum becomes active as well. In fact, some sound signals go directly to the cerebellum and bypass the auditory cortex completely. This was surprising, because until recently the cerebellum was thought to be mainly involved in movement and balance. This circuit may be important for connecting music to movements and emotions when we dance, because, as we now know, the cerebellum is also involved in emotion processing. When the cerebellum perceives order, we feel a certain sense of satisfaction, because the cerebellum is connected to the brain's reward centers. It also participates in the little surprises that music is always giving us, because once a rhythm or a pattern is established, our brains are not expecting a change. If the composer changes the pattern to something new, we are stimulated by the change, even excited, and this produces some of the thrill we derive from music.

Two other parts of the brain are involved in sound perception: the *hippocampus* and the *prefrontal cortex,* which govern different sorts of memory functions. In order to decipher a tune, your brain has to retain the notes it hears, along with all of their features, while it works to add these features together and recognize a pattern. The process, which is called *working memory,* takes place in the prefrontal cortex. Memories stored here are transient, and the trace lasts only as long as necessary for the brain to build the shape of the perception. Memories such as the ones we usually associate with the word "memory"—recollections of childhood, the recollection of what you had for lunch yesterday—are held in another part of the brain, called the *hippocampus* (the Greek word for "seahorse," since this is what its curly shape evoked in the minds of sixteenth-century anatomists). When you listen to a piece of music you heard long ago in high school, at the time you first fell in love, it can elicit the same emotions you associated with it at the prom, even if you're hearing it decades later. It is dipping into your hippocampus brain region and then triggering those emotions of infatuation and excitement. It is why the organ music Edward Searles listened to reminded him of his dead wife and brought forth all the feelings of love, happiness, and grief that were held in his memory.

How do the brain regions that control our many emotions link up with the complex process of healing? Can emotions heal? Before researchers could answer these questions, they had to develop technologies that could measure the brain's outflow pathways of emotion—the same pathways responsible for the goose bumps that so intrigued Dan Levitin. These are the nerve routes by which emotional responses are transmitted to the rest of the body, including the cells and organs of healing. Another musician-turned-scientist, by the name of Julian Thayer, chose to tackle this question.

Thayer often appears at medical conferences wearing a jacket and a black silk collarless shirt without a tie—hardly the usual conference attire. He looks more like a jazz musician than a famous psychophysiologist. In fact he is both, and his mathematical methods for analyzing complex heart-rate signals changed the way researchers interpret and measure the stress response. It took courage to follow this career path—courage that he came by through family experience. The family lore was that his grandparents lived so deep in the woods that they had to pump sunlight to them. It was only as an adult that Thayer realized why an African American man married to a white women had to live so far off the beaten path in the segregated South of the 1930s.

Thayer's own life was off the beaten path. He started out as a classical composer and double-bass player. He studied at the Berklee College of Music in Boston, but never finished his degree. He got side-tracked by hanging around at the Massachusetts Institute of Technology, across the river in Cambridge.

He had noticed that people listening to his musical compositions manifested a wide range of emotions. Like Levitin, he began to wonder whether music really could influence emotional responses. So he convinced one of his professors, the psychologist Robert Levenson (now at the University of California, Berkeley), to let him study people as they listened to music. After this research, he decided to take courses in psychology, music, and chemistry at Indiana University in Bloomington. Eventually, he got a Ph.D. in psychology. His first paper, based on that early research, was published in the *Journal of Psychomusicology* in 1983. It showed that music did indeed affect people's emotions, as well as other physiological responses such as heart rhythms.

The study was very cleverly designed. Thayer chose a silent movie and wrote two different musical scores for it—one stressful, the other relaxing. Then he showed it to a number of volunteer participants. In comparison to people who watched it with no sound at all, those who watched it with the stressful score showed signs of activation of their stress responses, and those who heard the relaxing score showed a calming effect. The music was clearly able to move the viewer's stress response in either direction, up or down. In 1980, when Thayer began his study, the methods for measuring the stress response in such settings were primitive. He was able to measure heart rate and skin conductance—a measure of sweating, used in lie-detector tests. But the more sophisticated measures of heart rhythms were just being developed.

Thayer realized that if he was to pursue such studies, he needed to find a method for obtaining precise measurements of the brain's responses to stress. He studied with a team of bioengineers in Italy, Alberto Malliani and Massimo Pagani, who were working on a way to measure the control of heartbeats by the nervous system. They attached small heart monitors to volunteers, in order to record heartbeats continuously over a period of twenty-four hours. The variability of the time intervals between beats was the key, because the rate of the heartbeats and the length of time between the beats are controlled by different parts of the nervous system. Malliani and Pagani reasoned that if they could develop an easily worn device which could accurately measure the interval between heartbeats, they could deduce, using mathematical formulas, which part of the nervous system was active and controlling the heart at any point in time. Over a three-year period, Thayer traveled back and forth to Milan to assist in the development of the new measurement technology.

These minute heart-rate variations, lasting only milliseconds, can now be measured and the pattern of variability can be calculated. When Thayer came into the field, researchers thought that only the input of adrenalin-like nerves could be measured with this technique. Adrenalin-like nerves and the chemicals they release speed up the heart and decrease the variability between beats. What Thayer discovered is that, by using complex mathematical analyses, he could also detect the contribution of the other nerve that wires the heart, the vagus nerve, which slows the heart by means of a nerve chemical called acetylcholine. This is part of the *parasympathetic* component of the nervous system, which acts like a brake when the adrenalin nerves of the *sympathetic* nervous system speed up the heart.

This experience persuaded Thayer to change careers (though he never gave up music entirely—he still plays double-bass in a jazz band). The research that he and his colleagues performed resulted in a device that you can carry around like an iPod in your pocket, but instead of listening to the rhythms of music, it listens to the rhythms of your heart and records the intervals between the beats. Such devices have made it possible to measure the activity of both components of the nervous system—the sympathetic (stress) part and the parasympathetic (relaxation) part—under all sorts of conditions.

Thayer went on to study the effects of different types of music on the nervous system, and many other studies have measured the effects of music on the heart. In every case, when music makes a person shift from a stress mode to a relaxed mode, the heart-rate variability shifts from the adrenalin-driven, sympathetic pattern to the more changeable pattern of the parasympathetic relaxation response.

There may be yet another reason we find some sounds and music calming and others jarring. It has to do with the same patterns we find visually calming—those infinitely repeating patterns found in nature called fractals. Ary Goldberger, who proposed that looking at fractals is pleasing to the human mind; proposed that the same may be true for listening to music.

Goldberger has shown that heart-rate variability patterns, which appear chaotic, can be analyzed mathematically and reduced to relatively simple equations. The more complex and variable a system, he pointed out, the healthier it is. He also showed that a body's complex rhythms can be analyzed and used as measures of health. These rhythms are akin to Julian Thayer's measures of heart-rate variability.

Goldberger likes to show his lecture audiences a series of graphic patterns, and ask them to pick the one they think looks healthiest and the one that looks the sickest. Often people choose the smoothest, least variable lines, or the ones with the most regular squiggles, as the healthier patterns. Goldberger, a short, quick man with twinkling eyes who proudly admits his resemblance to Groucho Marx, chortles at the response. This is exactly what he wants to hear because it is (to use an apt phrase) dead wrong. He points out that the condition in which there is the least variability in heart rate is death. In death, there are no rhythms at all—the body generates only straight lines. A desirable image is one in which variability is high. There are lots of squiggly lines oscillating around the horizontal, in what appears to be a chaotic pattern. This is the image of health.

If a note were assigned to each heart-rate interval, Goldberger wondered, would the music that resulted from these patterns be calming or jarring? He collaborated with his son (a musician, composer, and then medical student) to set heart-rate variability rhythms to music. They produced two CDs of soothing music based on healthy rhythms of the heart. The rhythms of sick hearts produced jarring sounds. Once again, it seems that when we are in sync with patterns that exist in nature, whether visual or auditory, we feel peaceful and calm.

Heart-rate variability and the adrenalin-like or acetylcholine vagus nerve impulses that control these rhythms are the endpoint of a long chain of events that occur after sounds hit your eardrums. It is through changes in these nerve pathways and the nerve chemicals they release that changes in the brain's emotion centers could affect the immune system and healing.

Can listening to music or to silence really help people heal? Logically, the answer should be yes, but few conclusive studies have been done. Many studies have looked at the effects of music on pain: pain during a medical procedure, pain after surgery, or the chronic pain of cancer. Overall, thousands of patients have been studied, and there is a great deal of variation in the results. Part of this variation may be due to the fact that many different conditions were lumped together. In one analysis, the effects of music on reducing pain intensity, while beneficial, were very slight: music reduced pain intensity by only about 0.4 on a scale of 1 to 10. Still, it caused some reduction in the dosage of opiate medication needed by patients—15 to 20 percent less, compared to the dosages needed by patients who did not listen to music. This is a small effect, if we consider that there was a 50 percent reduction of opiate dose in patients who were given additional nonopiate drugs and no music therapy. But from the patients' point of view, 20 percent is still substantial, especially if it means avoiding extra medication. If conditions are not lumped together, the results are more dramatic. Several Swedish studies have shown that patients undergoing hernia repair who listened to relaxing music while under anesthesia, or in the recovery room for one hour immediately after surgery, required significantly less morphine compared to patients who did not listen to music: one-third to one-half the dose. If something as simple and safe as listening to music can help lower the dosages of pain medication to this extent, it may indeed be a useful healer.

Even if adding music to the therapeutic environment may not alone bring about large effects on healing, simply eliminating loud noises that cause stress is sure to speed recovery. Stress has many deleterious effects on the immune system, prolonging wound healing, reducing the body's ability to make antibodies, and impairing the immune system's ability to fight infection in many other ways. It therefore stands to reason that removing loud, stressful sounds from a hospital environment could only be beneficial.

Enhancing the positive effects of sound should likewise help. Activating the vagus nerve, the way soothing music does, can affect the immune response. Kevin Tracey, a surgeon and researcher at the Feinstein Institute for Medical Research on Long Island, has shown that stimulating the vagus nerve electrically has rapid and profound effects on inflammation in the belly, suppressing an overactive immune response. We don't yet know if milder interventions (such as music), which turn on vagus nerve activity, are strong enough to affect the immune system as well. But it is possible that music could affect immune responses and healing through this very direct route.

Many studies do show that listening to music has measurable

effects on the production of certain antibodies in the saliva: the so-called *IgA antibodies,* which are the first line of defense in protecting against infection. Such research suggests that music can affect not only our emotions and the emotional outflow pathways of the brain, but also the ability of immune cells to fight infection.

It turns out, too, that singing can have profound effects on these same emotional and immune responses, but the effects differ with context. Amateur singers performing in a choir will experience a reduction in stress response and enhancement of mood; but professional singers, during stage performances, show an increase in stress response. In both cases, levels of IgA in saliva increase. In contrast, another immune molecule, which triggers inflammation, increases in professional singers along with the stress hormone cortisol. Both substances decrease in amateur singers. These studies tell us that, like everything else which affects ours moods and healing, individual experiences, memories, and expectations play a very important role.

Sound and silence have profound effects on the nervous system, on our emotional responses to the world around us, and on the nerve chemicals and hormones flowing from those emotion centers, which ultimately affect the immune system and how we heal. What about our other senses—those of touch and smell? Could these, too, contribute to healing?

4

COTTON WOOL AND CLOUDS OF FRANKINCENSE

Of all the ways in which we sense the world, touch and smell are the only two in which we come into direct contact with the things around us. This is obvious in the case of touch: you must run your fingers over a brick wall to feel its roughness, or sit on a stone bench to feel its hardness, or step into a bath to feel the warm water on your skin. But it's the same with smell. When you walk along a street in New York City and smell roasted peanuts, rotting garbage, grilled beef, and cooking oil, all mingled with diesel exhaust, you're coming into contact with tiny bits of those things. Or if you sit still upon a hillside on a breezy day, and smell a sequence of fresh-mown hay, manure, water from the lake, wet mud from the ditch, and pine trees mixed with honeysuckle, it is because each one has come to you, riding on the wind. In both cases, the air has brought you a few molecules of each substance, to sample with your nose.

The first thing that happens when you take an ordinary breath is that air enters your nostrils. As it heads toward the back of your throat, it flows past three fleshy shelves in the interior of your nose. Some of it also passes over a structure deep inside, hidden behind the topmost shelf, against the base of the skull. This is the *olfactory organ,* which detects odors. Its nerve cells, buried in a mucous membrane, send fibers up through a perforated patch of skullbone so thin that it is easily fractured. If the bone breaks, meningitis can set in, because the brain at that point is very close to the germ-filled outside world. But the patch of bone needs to be thin and perforated, so that the long fibers of the olfactory nerve cells have access to the brain.

When you sniff a flower, you take in more air than you do when breathing normally. The air flows and eddies past the olfactory organ. In mammals, a single sniff lasts in the range of 100–250 thousandths of a second, just enough time for the brain's olfactory centers to recognize and interpret the scent. Rats are better at this than people—they can accurately identify an odor in less than 100 thousandths of a second. But although humans are slower, they are remarkably good at detecting and distinguishing more than ten thousand odors, in vanishingly small amounts.

When you touch something, you feel its texture. This gives you a clue to what it might be, but it doesn't tell you what it is made of. When you smell something, you are identifying its chemical structure. The olfactory organ is an exquisitely sensitive chemical detector that can identify a substance on the basis of just a few molecules dissolved in air. Did you ever wonder why the air smells different on a warm summer evening after it has rained? The reason is that the drops of water coating everything—leaves, pavement, earth, grass—dissolve a little bit of these things, along with whatever is on their surface. As the water evaporates, molecules are released into the air in complex mixtures and you sense them through your olfactory organ. At various temperatures, different combinations of molecules dissolve in the water and are released into the air. So the air smells different on a spring day, in the heat of summer, and in midwinter. The air's scent can tell you the seasons, the time of day, and your location—countryside or city street, ocean beach or mountain lake. Gardenia, honeysuckle, orange blossom, and jasmine are all more pungent in the evening in summer. Fresh-mown grass and hay are summer, too. Wood burning in fireplaces is fall and winter.

Even if you have never been in southern Florida or along Italy's Amalfi Coast on a spring evening, you would immediately
recognize the odors of methyl anthranilate and geosmin. And
even if you had never received a dozen fragrant blooms on Val-
entine's Day, you would know two things about geranyl acetate:
that it is both related to and different from methyl anthranilate.
You would know that both scents are floral, and that they originate from two different kinds of flowers. Geranyl acetate is the
chemical that gives the rose its scent, and methyl anthranilate
comes from orange blossoms. Geosmin (literally, "earth smell")
is a tertiary alcohol that comes from algae and that gives wet
mud its scent. In 200 thousandths of a second, your nose and
brain can detect chemical differences and similarities among these
odors. The olfactory system registers smells much the same way
the visual system registers images and the auditory system registers sounds. First, the component features of the smell are detected; then the brain puts them together to form an olfactory
image of your surroundings.

When the molecules of odor hit the mucous membrane of
the olfactory organ, they dissolve in the mucous fluid around
the nerve cells and are carried along by capillary action according to their size. This is exactly how chemists assess the relative
size of molecules via *chromatography,* which operates on the
fact that chemicals of different weights and electrical charges
travel through water at different speeds. The larger, least soluble
ones—the ones with low electrical charges—travel slowest, and
the smaller, highly charged particles travel fastest.

When an odor molecule arrives at the olfactory organ, it
comes into contact with the olfactory nerve cells. These cells
have tiny *cilia* or hair-like structures which contain proteins of
different shapes. The proteins are the receptors for the odor
molecules. How can we possibly distinguish ten thousand odors?
How can we identify a scent in a flash of a second? Smell was the

last of the senses that scientists figured out. It seemed impossible that a single organ could possibly detect so many different odors so accurately, sensitively, and quickly.

The answer came in 1991, when Linda Buck and Richard Axel discovered a "super-family" of more than one thousand genes that determine our ability to detect and distinguish odors. In 2004 they received the Nobel Prize for their discovery. Most of these genes are active in rodents and other animals. Only about three hundred fifty are active in humans, but they suffice, with all of their permutations and combinations, to enable us to detect the full range of odors in our environment.

This large family of closely related genes produces a group of closely related proteins. Each protein folds into a slightly different configuration, and in the middle of its folds contains a tiny pocket with a unique shape. It can detect the presence of a single molecule of water, or a certain type of carbon atom, or a benzene ring with a particular orientation. It works because each scent molecule has precisely the right shape to fit the cleft.

Once the properly shaped odor molecule lands on one of these proteins, it binds tightly in its pocket, like a key within a lock. A molecule that doesn't fit will not bind—or if it fits imperfectly, it binds less tightly. Once it clicks into its spot, the molecule changes the shape of the receptor protein on which it sits, thus starting a cascade of biochemical events inside the cell: a channel forms in the cell surface, allowing electrically charged sodium and calcium atoms (ions) to enter; as they do so, the charge of the cell membrane changes, triggering an electrical impulse that travels to the nerve ending. This is the beginning of the transformation of a scent into electrical impulses in the brain.

The nose can detect not only the type of chemical it smells, but also the chemical's concentration. The lower the concentration—that is, the fewer the number of molecules dissolved in a given volume of air—the weaker the smell. The higher the concentration, the stronger the smell. The closer you are to the source of the smell, the more pungent it will be, because there are more molecules concentrated around its source. As the distance increases between you and the smell, the *concentration gradient* goes from high to low: the number of molecules decreases and the odor dissipates. Watch the puff of exhaust from a bus and you will see a dense cloud that gradually thins out as it floats away. You are watching the concentration gradient of the exhaust fumes. You can see these fumes because they consist of large particles, but the same happens with tiny molecules. The difference is that, with small molecules, you are perceiving the gradient with your nose instead of with your eyes.

When a dog follows a scent, it will follow the trail from weak to strong. The same is true for the wild pigs that sniff out truffles—those tasty French fungi that sell for hundreds of dollars per ounce. When the pigs pick up the scent, they will dig until they get to the source. Lobsters "sniff" the water with their antennae and can detect dissolved molecules. By comparing the concentrations detected by the two antennae, they can tell the direction the molecules are coming from and can trace them upstream until the concentration peaks. Our nostrils work the same way.

People—like dogs, rodents, pigs, and lobsters—smell in stereo. Each of our nostrils registers a slightly different concentration of an odor, and our brain can detect this infinitesimal difference. We can thus tell the direction the smell is coming from. People are much less skilled at this than dogs, which can easily pick up a scent and follow a trail. But scientists have shown that humans can be trained to do this, too.

A team comprising researchers from the University of California at Berkeley, Pennsylvania State University, and the Weizmann Institute in Israel dribbled essential oil of chocolate for ten meters through a grassy field, and tested whether people could follow the trail by scent. The thirty-two participants were not allowed to use any visual, auditory, or tactile cues—they were swathed in clothing, their eyes were masked, and their ears were covered. Crawling on hands and knees, twenty-one of the volunteers, nine women and twelve men, succeeded in tracking the scent on their first try. With nostrils blocked, they failed. The researchers then had two men and two women track the scent three times per day, three days per week, for two weeks. The participants improved dramatically in speed and accuracy with the training. They followed the same method that dogs use when tracking the scent of meat dragged over the ground: they sniffed repeatedly and zigzagged through the field. Though humans' nostrils are only about two centimeters apart, this is sufficient for people to detect slight differences in the concentration of a scent cloud, and thus provides information about the scent's location and source.

So as you go about your day, you encounter patches of scent that differ in shape and size and composition. Your perception of the intensity of each scent will vary not only with its concentration but also with the speed of your encounter—how quickly you move through the cloud. The information is coded in packets of nerve-cell firings that fit the duration of each sniff you take. The speed of electrical firing is also determined by the concentration of the substance in the air: the more concentrated the smell, the earlier and faster the nerve cells will fire. As a result, you gain a sense of both the chemical composition of your surroundings and the spatial distribution of each chemical in the air. Because the brain sorts these chemicals by individual features as well as by categories, you also know something about the family of fragrances that you encounter—whether they are floral, grassy, leafy, earthy, or briny; fishy or meaty; delicate or pungent; acrid or sweet. And in this way you form a 3-D image of the chemical composition of the world around you. Besides informing you about the chemical and physical landscape, your sense of smell also tells you about your social landscape—who is nearby, whether you find them attractive, and what dangers might be lurking beyond the range of your eyes and ears.

In downtown Philadelphia, a few blocks from the 30th Street Train Station, the urban landscape offers an amazing sight: an enormous golden statue of a nose! This ten-foot-high gilded sculpture includes a pair of full lips and part of a face, but has no eyes or ears. It looks like something one might find in an Egyptian tomb. Created in the 1980s by sculptor Arlene Love, it is a perfect symbol for the organization over which it presides: the Monell Chemical Senses Center, a research institute founded in 1968 and affiliated with the University of Pennsylvania. The center is entirely devoted to the study of smell and taste.

In the 1980s, Lewis Thomas—physician, cancer researcher, immunologist, poet, and philosopher of science—became the institute's board chairman. He had always had a particular interest in the phenomenon of smell. His father had been a country doctor. When Thomas was young, he had sometimes accompanied his father on visits to patients and had observed that smell was a very important part of the doctor's diagnostic toolkit. Prior to the early 1900s, doctors had only their noses as a means of detecting abnormal substances in body fluids. To test for diabetes, they would smell or even taste the patient's urine, to see if it was sweet. They would sniff the patient's breath; an acrid smell indicated excess lactic acid, a symptom of diabetic coma. The breath of a patient with pneumonia gave off the sickly sweet odor of certain kinds of bacteria. Even today, we use breathalyzers to detect excess alcohol. For early twentieth-century doctors, their noses were their breathalyzers.

Thomas was intrigued by the fact that dogs had such keen

powers of odor detection—that, for instance, police dogs could find a person from a single sniff of a shred of clothing. One thing particularly struck him, as an immunologist: a dog can tell any two people apart, unless they're identical twins. It's the same with the immune system, which makes no distinction between people who have the same genetic makeup. Identical twins can receive transplants of organs and tissues from each other without becoming ill. All the rest of us require extensive tests to find a compatible donor. The molecules that determine such a match are called *major histocompatibility* (MHC) molecules, and they are expressed on the surface of every cell. They are what give each individual, or each set of twins, a unique immunological identity. In his book *The Lives of a Cell* (1975), Thomas proposed that histocompatibility antigens might also be involved in our sense of smell. This theory turned out to be correct. Some fifteen years later, the researchers who proved it won the Nobel Prize.

At the same time, and independently, two researchers at the Memorial Sloan-Kettering Cancer Center, while breeding histocompatible mice for immunology research, noticed that male mice preferred to mate with a female who carried a different histocompatibility type. This observation and the Monell Center research that sprang from it proved what Thomas had postulated: that mammals do detect immune molecules through their nose. It is these molecules, excreted in the urine, that dogs sniff in order to tell which other dogs have marked the territory. Other molecules can also attract.

In his essay "A Fear of Pheromones," Lewis Thomas discussed the remarkable effect exerted by a female moth when it sprays the pheromone bombykol. *Pheromones* are small, fatty, odorless molecules that easily dissolve in air and are released from sweat glands near the hair follicles in animals. Pheromones are very powerful attractants to the opposite sex. It has been "soberly calculated," Lewis wrote, that if a female moth were to release "all the bombykol in her sac in a single spray, all at once, she could theoretically attract a trillion males in the instant." ("This is, of course," he noted wryly, "not done.") The organ that detects these vaporous compounds is the *vomeronasal complex*, which is located much closer to the nostrils than the olfactory organ and consists of two tiny pits on either side of the nasal septum with direct connections to the brain, including the parts of the brain that govern reproduction. In his essay, Thomas referred to a seminal paper that had been published the year before by a young Radcliffe student named Martha McClintock.

McClintock had noticed that all the women in her college dorm seemed to get their period at the same time. She published an article in *Nature* postulating that pheromones could be the cause of the synchronization of the menstrual cycle in women who room together. The phenomenon also occurs in female rodents housed in the same cage. McClintock went on to study this phenomenon in more detail, and in 1998 published another paper in *Nature* confirming and extending the original findings. She showed that in other species pheromones govern many behaviors, including mate preference, dominance relationships, and weaning.

Researchers at the Monell Center found that humans can detect the moods of those around them through their sense of smell. The study started out as a science project by a seventh-grader named Daniel McGuire, the son of one of the researchers. It was later replicated at the Monell Center laboratories and written up in the journal *Perceptual Motor Skills* by researchers Denise Chen and Jeannette Haviland-Jones. Twenty-five college-age men and women wore gauze pads under their arms while watching a fourteen-minute video that was either scary or funny. Forty women and thirty-seven men were then asked to smell the pads and report whether they thought the people who had provided the pads were afraid or happy. The participants identified the smell of pads worn during the frightening video as "scent of fear" more often than would be predicted by chance alone. Women proved to be much better at this task than men: they correctly identified both "fear odors" and "happy odors."

Although much research remains to be done on the way odors and volatile compounds secreted by our bodies relate to our moods, it is clear that these invisible compounds form an important part of our landscape and influence many physiological functions. How does our perception of chemicals in the air affect our bodies? Do scents have the power to heal?

Since the Middle Ages, pilgrims have walked the thousand-kilometer trail from the Tour St. Jacques in Paris, through the Massif Central in the heart of France, along the northern coast of Spain to the cathedral at Santiago de Compostela. The pilgrims took many routes, starting in various cities throughout western Europe, such as Frankfurt and Rome. Most passed through France, often through the town of Lourdes in the foothills of the Pyrenees. Others passed through Chartres, a town just outside of Paris. But when they crossed the Pyrenees, all converged on a single route: the Camino Frances ("French Way"). And all ended up in the town of Compostela, near the western tip of mainland Europe, a windswept ocean cliff called Finisterre, meaning "where the land ends" or "end of the world," as it surely seemed to be.

The pilgrims' goal was the shrine of Sant Iago (Saint James), who was an apostle of Jesus and whose remains, according to legend, were buried in the cathedral. Once the pilgrims arrived, filthy, wet, cold, and stinking from their long trek, they sought shelter in the church. They huddled on the floor and waited for the Mass to start. But before a word of prayer was uttered, six monks would hoist an enormous silver *botafumeiro*, or censer, high into the air on ropes. So heavy was the vessel that each monk was lifted up by his rope, as his confreres tugged on theirs. It was filled with frankincense, and its fragrant smoke would billow to the top of the cathedral's Gothic arches. As the censer rose slowly toward the ceiling, the monks would set it swinging in ever-increasing arcs, so that the sweet, spicy scent would drift down and settle upon the pilgrims below.

Today you can visit Santiago de Compostela and see the ritual practiced exactly as it has been for more than a thousand years. Catholic cathedrals around the world perform similar versions at Christmastime, but use much smaller, hand-held censers. As the bishop and the procession of clergy walk slowly down the aisle, a cloud of frankincense floats above them like a ghost, engulfing the congregation in its scent.

Until the Vatican II council in the 1960s, the frankincense ritual was performed daily as a blessing during the Mass and, on Christmas, was meant to evoke the gifts of the Magi. In twelfth-century Compostela, it was also aimed at cleansing the pilgrims of infectious diseases.

It is probably no accident that two of the three precious gifts that the Magi brought to the manger in Bethlehem were the fragrant resins myrrh and frankincense, which were known even in biblical times for their healing powers. They are extracted from small thorny bushes—the *Boswellia* and *Commiphora* species of the *Burseraceae* family—which grow in South Asia, the Middle East, and Africa, especially Somalia, Ethiopia, and Kenya. The *Boswellia* plant, from which frankincense is extracted, grows in India and around the Red Sea. The chemical composition of these plants differs according to climate and location. Their country of origin is thus revealed by their chemical profile. The Queen of Sheba was said to have brought King Solomon the closely related balsam tree, whose thickened gum is known as *balm*. He cultivated the trees in Judea. Their healing virtue is referred to in Jeremiah 8:22: "Is there no balm in Gilead? Is there no physician there? Why then is not the health of the daughter of my people recovered?" The Romans considered balm so precious that when they conquered Judea, they carried saplings back to Rome and guarded them with sentries.

All three of these resins exude a balsamy odor and have served throughout history as perfumes. Myrrh and balm were used to treat wounds—Greek soldiers carried myrrh into battle. Frankincense was said to ease labored breathing in asthma, soothe colds and bronchitis, and help remove scars.

Frankincense and myrrh come in several forms: a water-soluble gum, an alcohol-soluble resin, and various oils. They contain a mixture of dozens of small molecules, including steroid-like molecules that evaporate easily and have a spicy smell. Some studies have shown that frankincense, when added to immune cells, can enhance their activity or reduce inflammation. Other studies have shown that it has antifungal and antibacterial effects. So the monks of Santiago de Compostela were likely right to bathe the tired and sickly pilgrims in soothing clouds of frankincense.

Many other fragrant oils have been known, since ancient times, to have healing properties. When King David, in the Twenty-Third Psalm, says, "Thou anointest my head with oil," he is probably referring to an oil that is both sacred and healing. In biblical times, holy oil was often a blend of olive oil, sweet spices, myrrh, and frankincense, "compounded after the art of the apothecary" (Exodus 30:23–35). Healing the soul and healing the body went together: holy oil represented divine blessing, which would drive out pernicious influences, demons, disease. Oils of lavender, sandalwood, tea tree, eucalyptus, geranium, and chamomile have also been used for their antibacterial effects. Joseph Lister, the first physician to advocate antisepsis during surgery, used oil of thyme to cleanse wounds.

Employing scented oils in the treatment of illness is called *aromatherapy*. It is based in large part on historical references and the age-old practice, in both Western and Eastern cultures, of using such oils for healing. Recent pharmacological research has shown that some of these oils are effective, alone or in combination, against specific strains of bacteria. In one study, a combination of grapefruit seed extract and geranium oil killed antibiotic-resistant and antibiotic-sensitive *Staphylococcus;* lavender, tea tree, and patchouli oil also had some effect. This area of research is clearly ripe for study, and should yield important new compounds for treating wounds, infection, and inflammation.

Fragrant oils have not only been applied to wounds and diseased skin, but have also been inhaled for their healing effects on mood. Florence Nightingale moistened the foreheads of wounded soldiers with lavender oil, which is said to have a relaxing effect and is often used at nighttime as a sedative. Other essential oils that are said to reduce stress are chamomile, geranium, rose, sweet marjoram, and valerian.

It is difficult to design accurate, controlled studies for testing how and under what conditions these compounds might work, because their odors are so recognizable. Until recently, most publications relied on individual reports—known as *anecdotal evidence* or *testimonials*—or on studies in which the effects of the active compound were not compared to those of other compounds.

Several studies suggest that fragrant oils such as lavender can indeed ease tension, improve mood, and induce sleep. One experiment showed that in rats with an intact sense of smell, inhalation of valerian and rose scents prolonged sleep that had been induced by pentobarbital, while lemon odor shortened it. Brain electrical activity in these rats, measured by electroencephalogram (EEG), also changed accordingly. In contrast, rats who had lost their sense of smell showed no effect. The experiment thus provided evidence that it was indeed the smell of these compounds which prolonged sleep.

Another study, focusing on ten men and ten women, showed that, compared to sweet almond oil, lavender oil helped to treat mild insomnia. EEG changes have also been shown in people inhaling lavender oil, with shifts toward patterns characteristic of positive moods. Lavender also decreased memory and reaction times, as would be expected in a compound that causes drowsiness. In a study in which people's moods and EEG were examined, lavender and chamomile made the participants feel comfortable, while sandalwood reduced their comfort. At the same time, among people smelling lavender and chamomile, the EEG awake-pattern alpha-1 brain waves decreased, especially in the parietal and temporal lobes, the brain regions involved in processing smells and other sense-data. But other studies have shown *increases* in EEG alpha-1 pattern, showing how difficult it is to perform these studies and compare them under different conditions.

Some studies have measured skin and hormonal stress reactions to inhaled odor molecules. Valerian can decrease the levels of the stress hormone cortisol, as well as decrease contact hypersensitivity reactions in the skin, possibly by reducing levels of certain immune molecules that cause inflammation. Though only small numbers of people have been studied, these findings suggest that such aromatic compounds might benefit healing of both body and mood.

One reason it is difficult to compare the effects of fragrances on mood is that they are powerful at triggering memories. Yet this very feature could also amplify their healing effects. Our sense of smell develops early and is linked indelibly to memory. Perhaps this has to do with the way an infant first experiences the world, through the smell and taste of its mother's milk. You can find your way back to comfort, to times in childhood when all was safe, through the power of certain scents—the smell of balsam at Christmastime, fudge and chicken soup in Grandma's kitchen, brand new dolls, or birchwood baseball bats. People from other cultures will have different triggers for childhood memories—perhaps the scent of curry, fried samosas, ginger mixed with soy, cooked rice, or fried plantain. Even powerful unpleasant smells, if strongly associated with a positive emotion, can transport a person back to the past. There is an Asian fruit called the durian which, when cut open, emits the smell of rotting flesh, though its taste is very sweet. Those who have grown up eating it will crave it, wherever they are in the world, because it reminds them of home. Those who have never encountered it will be sickened by it, unable even to venture a taste.

Researchers at the Monell Center have found that such emotional associations vary markedly with the individual and are culturally dependent. In their studies, they infuse minute amounts of different odor molecules into a sealed room in which temperature, humidity, and lighting are all controlled. The participants are seated in front of a computer, and are monitored with cameras so that the experimenters can note their reactions. They are connected to all sorts of physiological instruments, including heart-rate and breath-rate monitors, and they are given questionnaires that assess their moods and feelings. Sometimes the researchers measure exhaled gases, in order to detect molecules which increase during inflammation. In this way, physiological and emotional reactions to tiny amounts of odor molecules can be measured in real time. It is clear from such studies that individual experience, much of it based on memory, plays a vital part in the reactions.

Repeated association of a scent with a mood can firmly link the two, the same way a color can become linked with a mood: through the Pavlovian process of conditioning. This can happen after many repeated exposures, or—if the emotion is powerful enough—it can happen in a millisecond. Once such a feeling, whether good or bad, becomes attached to a sense-perception through memory, the two are very hard to pry apart.

Touch, likewise, can be irrevocably bonded to emotions from earliest childhood. The way your mother may have soothed your burning forehead during a childhood illness will continue to soothe and calm you throughout your life, even if later touches come from another person. Especially in small mammals, a mother's touch is essential for survival, for the warmth it provides. Newborn rodent pups, when separated from their mothers for just a few minutes, show a large increase in their stress response, which can be partly reversed by placing them on a heating pad set to body temperature.

In the 1960s and 1970s, when new technologies were being introduced into neonatal intensive-care units (NICUs), excess touching of the tiny infants was prohibited, largely for fear of infection. But Tiffany Field, a psychologist and researcher at the University of Miami, changed all that.

Field noticed that when she massaged her own baby daughter, who had been born prematurely, the baby's stress behaviors immediately and perceptibly diminished. Field then set out to prove that touching premature infants would be beneficial to their health. At first she encountered resistance: doctors and nurses who ran the neonatal intensive-care units were so focused on stabilizing and maintaining the babies' condition, that touch was the last thing they were interested in. It seemed like hocus-pocus, soft science, even potentially dangerous.

But Field persisted. She developed a standardized method of massage, which included gently stroking the arms, legs, back, chest, and tummy, as well as gently flexing and rotating the limbs—a sort of passive Pilates routine. She did this for three fifteen-minute periods per day. She then performed studies in which she documented the babies' growth, food intake, and nutritional status, which are the most important measures of overall health. An ailing infant will not eat; it will lose weight and fail to thrive.

Field found dramatic growth increases in the infants who were stroked, compared to those who received minimal touching. After only five days of massage therapy, the babies had gained a daily average of 53 percent more weight, compared to the babies who were cared for under the minimal-touch policy. They also slept less—a sign of physical maturation in preemies, who tend to sleep much longer than full-term infants. Field went on to study the reasons for this. Because the babies were already being monitored for all sorts of physiological responses, she was able to measure many of these, including activity of the vagus nerve, which shifts heart-rate variability away from a stress pattern and toward a relaxation pattern. This nerve also enhances stomach contractions and digestion.

Field found that in the babies who were massaged, vagus nerve tone and stomach contractions increased. She thus proved beyond a shadow of a doubt that touch therapy is good for infants' health, and also how it works. Her studies convinced the medical community that massage should be included in the daily medical care of premature infants. Although some NICUs still maintain a minimal-touch policy, an increasing number of hospitals—close to 40 percent surveyed in 2003, and even more today—have instituted massage therapy as a regular part of their treatment regime. In 1992 Field set up the Touch Research Institute in Miami, where massage and touch therapy are now being used to treat many conditions, including pain, stress, depression, and unexplained wasting in the elderly.

Touch tells us a great deal about the world around us, in a much more fine-grained way than other senses. You need to be close to an object in order to touch it, to feel its texture, moisture, and temperature.

When you touch something, the pressure receptors in your skin tell you how hard you are pressing. These receptors, called *mechanoreceptors,* are present in virtually every living cell. Bacteria have mechanoreceptors in their cell membranes; this is how they sense the world and "know" when they are bumping up against other bacteria. These tiny transducers, consisting of just a few molecules, lie within the membrane of the cell and respond to pressure. As pressure deforms the cell membrane, channels in the mechanoreceptors are also deformed, and open up to allow charged atoms into the cell. The flow of these ions creates an electrical current.

In multicelled animals, from fruit flies to rodents to humans, it is this electrical current which signals the brain. In mammals, the deformation of the channels by pressure and touch occurs in a variety of tiny organs embedded in the skin. Some are called *Meissner's corpuscles,* others *Pacinian corpuscles* or *neurites,* depending on their structure and location. Meissner's corpuscles are swellings in the long nerve fibers in the skin; Pacinian corpuscles are located at the ends of long fibers of nerves whose cell bodies lie in the spinal cord; and neurites have long extensions and spikes that are thought to be sensitive to mechanical deformation. These pressure-sensing organs all work the same way: pressure deforms channels, causing ions to flow into the cell. The electrical current that results is carried along nerve pathways to the brain.

The ion channels that make possible our sense of touch are exquisitely sensitive to a vast range of pressures, spanning more than eight orders of magnitude. This is why you can feel the fuzz on a peach, the softness of moss, the roughness of a granite boulder, or the smoothness of a marble tile. It is why, when you walk barefoot on the beach, you can tell whether you are walking on sand or pebbles or a wooden boardwalk.

This is also the way hearing works, though in hearing the mechanical deformation that disturbs the hair cells in the cochlea is caused by puffs of air. As in touch organs, the hair cells are tethered to ion channels, which open in response to the movement of the hair, triggering electrical impulses in the auditory nerve and eventually leading to the perception of sound.

The sense of touch is also connected to our sense of sight. When you look at a plank of wood, you can tell whether it is likely to feel rough or smooth, and you make this judgment on the basis of its light-reflecting characteristics. The ability to make such judgments is probably learned. But blind people, even those blind from birth, are very adept at drawing pictures of what they "see" by touch. Just as sighted people primarily see edges, blind people likewise sense edges through touch. When researchers at the University of Toronto asked blind people to draw what they perceived by touch, their sketches were very similar to those of sighted people: they used outlines to mark edges, and contours and converging lines to convey distance and perspective. This ability to form an image of an object through the sense of touch is called our *haptic sense*.

Thus, we use vision, hearing, smell, and touch to gather information about our surroundings. Each sense detects individual features of what we perceive. Our brains then integrate these features in time and space to create a three-dimensional, richly colored, stereophonic, and scented image that tells us where we are. The sense-pictures change constantly as the world alters around us at every moment of our lives. And in response, the brain continuously uploads the new information and incorporates it into constantly revised versions of our world.

What happens when we move around? Does moving through our environment, rather than just passively viewing it, have a different impact on us? Can it trigger feelings of fear and stress, or a sense of calm? Does it change how we feel and how we heal?

5

MAZES AND LABYRINTHS

When Harry Potter enters the maze during the Triwizard Tournament in *The Goblet of Fire,* his nerves, his self-confidence, and his senses are immediately put under enormous strain. The "towering hedges cast black shadows across the path and . . . they were so tall and thick . . . [that] the sound of the surrounding crowd was silenced." He can see nothing ahead of him, and the "maze was growing darker with every passing minute as the sky overhead deepened to navy." As he searches for a way through, he is repeatedly faced with choices. Which direction should he take? How dangerous is each enchanted creature he confronts? What spell should he use to combat its powers? He hears his fellow competitors gaining fast upon him, and has no time to dawdle. We can feel the "clammy coldness stealing over him" as if it were our own. We can feel his terror, his "heart hammering," the "blood pounding in his ears."

What Harry is experiencing is his body's response to stress. And we understand how he feels—because even though we have never been in an enchanted maze, we have all experienced the stress response at some point in our lives.

In an article published in *Nature* in 1936, physician and scientist Hans Selye first used the word "stress" in its current sense: the body's nonspecific response to an external demand. Although Selye is often credited as the first author of the term as we know it, both the word and the concept had been around for a very long time. The ancient Romans used a word with a similar meaning—*stringere,* "to squeeze tight," "graze," "touch," or "injure." When the word entered the English language in the fourteenth century, it continued to refer to physical hardships of the environment. By the nineteenth century, the word had begun to take on a meaning combining the environment's physical effects with the body's responses to them. Then, in 1934, physiologist Walter B. Cannon showed that animals produce adrenalin in response to such stresses. This was indeed the first proof that the physical environment could trigger a bodily response. Selye took the concept one step further, showing that many other hormones were produced in response to stress, and that these could have lasting physical consequences on the body.

Selye was so passionate about this idea that he traveled the world to push for its acceptance. He succeeded: the word "stress" has made its way into virtually every language across the globe. So convinced was Selye of the importance of his theories, that he carved the structure of the stress hormone cortisol into the keystone above his front door and another atop a column in McGill University's old Anatomy Building. It was said that when he carved the former, his wife held him by the legs as he hung upside down with hammer and chisel. For the latter, he climbed a tall ladder to carve it in the dark of night. This piece of embarrassing graffiti had been hidden until the paint with which university authorities quickly covered it more than fifty years ago finally began to peel. His almost evangelical insistence on his theories and the grandiosity with which he pursued his mission alienated his colleagues, whose whispered dinner-table conversations about him often switched to foreign tongues, so that children within earshot couldn't repeat any disparaging remarks. My father was one of those colleagues, and my sister and I were two of those children. Some of this irritation may have stemmed from envy, but Selye had committed an even graver sin than self-promotion. Instead of talking only to his colleagues and using scientific jargon, he had the temerity to talk to the lay press and the public in clear, accessible language. And his ideas caught on. He became a widely known figure, even appearing in ads in *Reader's Digest*. The more popular he became, the more his colleagues shunned him.

At the same time, he had a loyal and devoted following of students. I remember, as a child, watching him from the shadows as he marched confidently down the hallway by his laboratories, a gaggle of adoring and intent students in tow. One of them, Roger Guillemin, went on to win the 1977 Nobel Prize in Physiology and Medicine for his discoveries of the hormones of the brain's stress center, the hypothalamus.

In 1936, Selye had emigrated from Austria to Canada, where he taught at McGill and then at the Université de Montréal. In the decades prior to his death in 1982, he trained generations of students, many of whom became professors at institutions all across the United States and Canada. By the centennial of his birth, in 2007, the academic community no longer felt the need to distance itself from Selye, his unconventional ideas, and his flamboyant ways. For it turned out that he was largely right. His theories about the brain's stress response were eventually proven by carefully designed experiments. We now know that the body and brain release specific hormones and chemicals when under stress. His idea that these responses could affect the immune system and make an organism sick also turned out to be true.

Yet the stress response is not as nonspecific as Selye had thought. There are many kinds of stress—physical, psychological, physiological—and there are many different nerve pathways by which the brain responds to these demands. When exposed to a stressful event, the hypothalamus starts pumping out the brain's stress hormone, *corticotropin releasing hormone* (CRH).

This in turn makes the pituitary gland, which hangs just beneath the brain on a slender stalk, pump out *adrenocorticotropic hormone* (ACTH). This hormone travels through the bloodstream to the adrenal glands, which sit atop the kidneys, and makes them pump out *cortisol,* a hormone that is similar to the drug cortisone.

It was a student of Roger Guillemin's, the chemist Jean Rivier, along with his colleague Wylie Vale and two others from the Salk Institute, who finally solved the structure of CRH. They called it *corticotropin releasing factor* (CRF), because it had not yet been identified as a hormone and because it had many other activities in the brain. In 1955, Guillemin had published a paper showing that an extract of hypothalamic tissue from sheep could stimulate the pituitary to release ACTH, but he had been unable to characterize the chemical that did this. One reason was that there was so little of it; in those days, large quantities of source material were needed before scientists could purify and identify proteins. In order to carry out the chemical analyses, the researchers pooled hypothalamic tissue from 490,000 sheep—material that was being discarded by butchers. The brain's stress hormone turned out to be a small protein, called a *peptide,* made up of a string of only forty-one amino acids. So small and yet so powerful!

When the brain's stress-hormone axis kicks into gear, nerve cells in a region deep inside the brain stem start firing quickly, releasing an adrenalin-like nerve chemical called *norepinephrine.* This part of the brain is called the *locus ceruleus,* Latin for "blue spot," because that's what it looked like to sixteenth-century anatomists. The brain's fear center, the amygdala, also becomes active. Then the adrenal glands and the adrenalin-like "sympathetic" nerves release adrenalin and related nerve chemicals. It is these hormones and nerve chemicals, acting together, that make you feel stressed. These are what affect Harry Potter as he enters the maze, making his heart pound, his skin clammy, his thoughts anxious.

You too can have this experience if you visit the boxwood-hedge maze at Hampton Court Palace on the Thames River, just outside London. Built for William III in 1606, the maze was created to entertain the lords and ladies of the court. The hedges, with their faintly cat-urine, antique sort of smell, are more than eight feet tall, so once you are inside the maze, you cannot see out. You can hear muffled giggling and squealing as others try to find their way, but you can't see them. Your only escape is to try different paths and hope they don't lead to dead ends. At first this is fun, but the more often you try a path that leads nowhere, the more anxious you become, especially if dusk is falling and closing time is approaching. You might easily begin to imagine supernatural creatures lurking in the shadows, and, more realistically you may fear being stuck in the maze all night.

What is it about mazes that triggers anxiety and the stress response? Two important features are responsible, and they involve the senses that are most important in finding your way: vision and hearing. In a maze, you cannot see where you are going and there are no clear sounds to guide you. Without full use of these two senses, you become disoriented.

Furthermore, a maze continually presents you with disturbing choices, dead ends, and new territories. You do not know how long the solution will take or how many twists and turns will get you out. Choices, uncertainty, and novelty are all potent triggers of the stress response. Place an animal in a new cage and stress centers in the brain immediately become active. A new environment is likewise a powerful trigger of the stress response in humans. Think of how you feel when you move into a new house, or on the first day of classes in a new school, or when you move to a new city. It takes days or even weeks to become accustomed to the place, so that it no longer seems strange and frightening.

The two together, a new environment and impaired vision, amplify anxiety and the stress response. Raise the bar yet again and add many different choice points, and anxiety will increase even more. Add another variable (diminished light) and even another (elevation above the ground) and, if the organism being tested is a rat, it will freeze at the points that offer the most frightening combination of choices.

Replicas of the Hampton Court maze were used as early as 1901 in studies of rat and primate behavior. Early researchers found that rats and monkeys could, with practice, learn to negotiate the maze. Such environments are now routinely used in preclinical testing of the efficacy of anti-anxiety drugs. A much simpler version of the Hampton Court maze, consisting of just two crossed arms, is called an *elevated plus maze,* because it is shaped like a plus sign and is raised about two feet off the ground. In rodents, this structure triggers anxiety behaviors and stress responses, including freezing, increased defecation (measured by the number of fecal pellets the rat leaves in its path), and elevations of the rat's equivalent of cortisol in its blood.

Unpleasant as these reactions may seem, if the rat in the maze had no stress response, it would fail to survive in the real world. It is the stress response that helps Harry Potter marshal his strength and maintain his focus, enabling him to continue on his quest. While it is bad to have too much of a stress response, which makes you freeze, it is also bad to have too little in times of danger. If Harry failed to be vigilant and were unable to concentrate on the task at hand, if he sat down in the maze and went to sleep, he'd be carried off by the next skrewt that came along. Similarly, if a rat or mouse in the wild were to fall asleep in a new environment, it would very likely be eaten by a predator. Our stress response is essential—to focus our attention, maintain our vigilance, help us to perform at peak, and give us the energy to fight or flee. In a novel environment, your stress response will help you notice details necessary for your escape or for finding your way. These are life-saving behaviors that are needed for survival. This is why all animals—insects, fish, birds, mice, humans—all have a stress response. Without it, the individual and the species would not survive. The stress response becomes counterproductive only when it is extreme. That's when it hinders your escape and impairs your performance.

This is because there is a *dose effect* of stress on performance, described by an "inverted U-shaped curve." Imagine an upside-down U, a curve shaped like a rainbow. The farther to the right you move on the curve, the more stressed you are; the higher up on the curve you are, the better your performance on a given task. At the far left end of the rainbow, you are completely relaxed, perhaps half-asleep and dozing. At this point, you are not performing much—you wouldn't be driving a car or writing a report or taking an exam. You certainly would not be able to negotiate your way through a maze. But move to the middle and top of the rainbow, to a point where your stress response is turned on just enough, and you are performing at your peak. You can feel the juices flowing and you feel excited, competent, and productive. Move to the far right end of the rainbow, where your stress response is at a maximum, and your performance falters. You slide down the edge of the curve and, like a rat, freeze in your tracks. If you're speaking in front of an audience, this is where you choke and are unable to say a word.

Gary Aston-Jones, a neuroscientist at the University of Pennsylvania, solved the puzzle of why this should be. He studied a number of monkeys, inserting electrodes into their locus ceruleus—the area in the brain stem that governs vigilance, focused attention, and the adrenalin component of the stress response. Once the electrodes were in place, the monkeys went about their usual routine while Aston-Jones monitored the nerve-cell activity in that tiny region of the brain. When the monkeys were completely relaxed and dozing, there was very little nerve-cell firing. When they were concentrating on a task they had learned—say, pressing a lever to get a pellet of food— individual nerve cells started to fire a lot. When they became stressed, all the nerve cells in that brain area began firing indiscriminately. This is when the monkeys' performance failed.

Think of email spam. Receive a few emails and you have useful information. Receive massive amounts of email all at once, and your server jams up. The only thing to do is clear out the spam, shut down, and reboot. We understand this about our computers, but not about ourselves. We need to learn when to shut down and go offline, literally and figuratively, to rest and recuperate. But the goal is not to be relaxed all the time. If you're ready to sleep, you want your stress response to be tuned low. But when you need to perform at your best or get out of danger, you need your stress response to be tuned up and working for you. The goal is for your stress response to be appropriately activated for the task at hand—to always find the middle of your rainbow.

One of the things that affects stress levels is the degree of control you have over a situation. The more you are in control, the less stressed you will be; the rush of hormones and nerve chemicals will make you feel stimulated, even exhilarated. The less control you have, the more stressed you feel. In a maze, you have no control over the twists and turns and dead ends you encounter, and this causes tension and anxiety.

Part of the trick to reducing the stress response is to fool your brain into thinking you have some degree of control. One anti-stress buffer that can bring you back to balance, especially in new environments and novel situations, is practice. Each time you walk through a maze, the stress reaction lessens until eventually it disappears. You have learned each twist and turn, and you don't have to make choices at each step. The route is no longer new. The more familiar places are, the less likely they are to trigger anxiety and the stress response. This is what happens when you move to a new city and drive around for the first time. A map might help, but you will still feel anxious and you might lose your way once or twice. Eventually, with practice, you no longer need the map and can navigate the route without anxiety.

Mazes have always been associated with fear and stress, from the time maze-like designs first appeared, in Greece, around 320 to 140 B.C.E.—the period between the death of Alexander the Great and the annexation of Greece by Rome. A famous example is described in the Cretan myth of the Minotaur, where it is called a labyrinth. Actually, labyrinths and mazes have very different structures.

Unlike a maze, with many choice points and many paths, a true labyrinth has only one path in and one path out. The one in leads to the center, and the one out leads back to the starting point. There are no decisions to be made and no blind alleys, and, most important, you can see the path ahead. There is no reason to be vigilant—you simply follow the path. Unlike a maze, a labyrinth does not inspire fear or the stress response. It calms.

The Roman scholar Pliny (24–79 C.E.) and the Greek philosopher Plutarch (45–120 C.E.) wrote about the Minoan labyrinth. They described it as a fearful thing, in which unlucky souls routinely lost their way and were devoured by the beast that lived within it. This description fits a maze better than it fits a labyrinth, but by the time they wrote, these scholars were relying on long-lost hearsay accounts. So whether this structure actually existed, and precisely what it was, is still a mystery.

The story goes that King Minos, the ruler of ancient Crete, had an enormous labyrinth built under his palace. The artist and

architect Daedalus was its designer. At its center, the king kept a
monstrous beast: the Minotaur. Half-human and half-bull, this
creature devoured any living thing that ventured near its lair. It
was the offspring of an illicit union resulting from a curse that
caused King Minos' wife, Pasiphaë, to fall in love with a beautiful white bull sent from the sea by the god Poseidon.

King Minos used the Minotaur to wreak revenge, and to
terrorize peoples he defeated in war. In order to punish the
Athenians for the death of one of his sons, Minos extracted a
tribute: he forced the Athenians to send seven maidens and
seven warriors to be sacrificed to the Minotaur. According to the
myth, the youths and maidens would wander around for days,
lost in the labyrinth, until devoured by the Minotaur. One day,
Theseus, son of the Athenian king, Aegeus, vowed to travel to
Crete to slay the Minotaur. When Theseus arrived in Crete,
Minos' daughter Ariadne fell instantly in love with him and con-
trived to help him. She gave him a ball of twine to unroll behind
him as he walked deeper into the labyrinth. The prince found
his way to the Minotaur and killed the monster, then followed
the string all the way back through the winding passageways to
freedom.

Today you can visit King Minos' palace at Knossos, just outside the city of Heraklion on Crete. The archaeological site has
been partly reconstructed, with blood-orange walls, fat lotus-
shaped pillars, murals of turquoise dolphins, and frescoes of
nubile, bare-breasted maidens doing back-flips over the horns
of bulls. You can wander through the expanse of halls, thinking of the awe that this place must have inspired in all who entered. Even today the maze of paths and the number of rooms
are so extensive that without a guide you would probably get
lost. According to legend, the Minotaur's lair was beneath the
palace, but no such place has ever been found. Still, you can eas-

ily imagine the visceral fear of those who tried to find their way through these corridors, fearing that a wild beast might be lurking around every bend.

No one knows when the first true labyrinths were built, but it seems that they have existed throughout history. Pliny's *Natural History,* containing a catalogue of all known labyrinths in the ancient world, became a standard source on the subject from its publication around 50 C.E. to the Middle Ages. The most famous medieval labyrinth still extant is the one created in 1260 in the cathedral at Chartres, a short distance from Paris. This labyrinth, like others of its type, has no walls. It is composed of a single continuous winding path set into the cathedral's floor in colored stone. Labyrinths typically have seven circuits, forming a pattern that resembles a multi-petaled flower. That is, the path winds around seven times before reaching the center, and then winds around again in overlapping circuits to reach the single exit, next to the starting point.

Remains of labyrinth-like structures can be found all over Scandinavia and northern Europe, where they are often made of loosely placed rocks lined up in the characteristic pattern. They are also found in classical Roman floor mosaics all around the Mediterranean—in Spain, France, Italy, Greece, Cyprus, and along the coast of North Africa. There is even one scratched like graffiti on a doorpost in Pompeii. In Britain, ancient labyrinth designs have been cut into turf, and can be found in England, northern Wales, Ireland, and as far north as Scotland. There are labyrinths carved in stone in petroglyphs dating as far back as 3000 B.C.E. and in Bronze Age tombs in Sardinia, northwest Spain, and Cornwall. Medieval labyrinths, like the one at Chartres, are found in churches across England, France, Germany, and Italy, with the majority in northern France and southern England. Many depict Theseus and the Minotaur at their center. But the labyrinth design is not unique to Europe. It has also been found in India, Afghanistan, Java, Sumatra, and the New World, at sites left by the Pueblo Indians, the Hopi, the Zuni, and others.

Why are these structures so widespread? What purpose did they serve, and who put them there? Theories abound. The axes of some labyrinths, including the one at Chartres, have such a clear relationship to the sun and the movement of celestial bodies, that some scholars think these structures were ancient astronomical charts.

The Chartres labyrinth lies just beneath the cathedral's rose window, in front of the western entrance. If you visit the cathedral close to the summer solstice, you will see an amazing sight: a sunbeam moving slowly along the labyrinth's path. At noon on June 21, the date of the solstice, it falls directly on a nail head that has been placed in the floor. Although this was a later addition in the case of Chartres, many other labyrinth-like structures do have features that would lend themselves to astronomical functions.

Yet beyond their possible use as solar clocks, another interpretation has suggested that labyrinths were never meant to be vertical structures at all. Some scholars believe that the labyrinth's winding path, known as "Ariadne's thread," actually marked the steps of a dance. There is much to be said for this interpretation, as descriptions of dances that follow this pattern exist in ancient literature. All are rites of passage, often called the Game of Troy. These involve young men who prove themselves as warriors, or young men and women who perform the dance as an initiation and fertility ritual. Indeed, one Etruscan vase dating to 600 B.C.E. depicts this in X-rated graphic form. On one side is a line of young beardless warriors marching in single file on foot and then astride horses, next to a labyrinth. On the other are two couples, long black hair flowing, both completely naked and anatomically correct. In each image, the female lies on her back in a different erotic position, with the male atop her, copulating. This might be why for centuries the Catholic church viewed these designs, inlaid in stone in their greatest cathedrals, with some suspicion as heathen artifacts and even tried to cover them up.

A dance-like form and purpose would fit the effect that labyrinths have on the movement and mood of all who enter them. A labyrinth draws you in and leads you on a single, gentle, calming path. It is calming because it forces you to focus your attention step by step on the way in front of you and on your inner thoughts, and drains your mind of all else. It makes you walk slowly as you wend your way around. There is something intrinsically soothing in this ritual.

And there is another calming effect that labyrinths exert on the visitor. It has to do with one of the tricks Harry Potter uses to control his stress response when it seems to be getting the better of him: "He took a deep, steadying breath, then got up again and hurried forward." Walking a labyrinth makes you breathe slowly in rhythm with your pace.

Slow, steady breathing is a very effective way to manage the stress response. This is because it activates the vagus nerve that counters the adrenalin-like sympathetic nervous-system response. During cardiopulmonary resuscitation, when a person's heart and breathing have stopped, strict guidelines tell rescuers how many times to compress the chest and administer restorative breaths. These guidelines have changed over the years, because it turns out that rescuers were giving breaths too often and patients were dying from hyperventilation. Resuscitation guidelines now advise that rescuers should give one breath every six to seven seconds once the heart has started up again. One breath every six to seven seconds: try counting that, while breathing in and breathing out. It seems incredibly slow, but this is the pace that provides the optimum amount of oxygen and carbon dioxide to nourish the tissues and keep the brain working well. It also calls into play the vagus nerve, the same nerve that calms the rhythms of the heart.

Walking a labyrinth, where all you need to do is concentrate on the path ahead and breathe in rhythm with your steps, can slow your breathing if you are anxious and allay the brain's drive toward anxiety. All walking meditations call for regular breathing. As your breathing drops to a comfortable pace, your heart rate downshifts to match, and calm prevails. This is precisely what coping techniques such as meditation, yoga, Tai Chi, and walking meditations all do. They move you back toward the middle of your rainbow—away from the extremes of stress that impair performance, and toward a point that is optimal for the task at hand. One of the ways they do this is through breathing.

Two Harvard cardiologists were among the first to tackle the connection between breathing and relaxation in a scientific way. One was Ary Goldberger, the researcher who studied heart-rate variability and related its patterns to soothing music. The other was Herbert Benson, who for many years studied mind-body interventions, particularly meditation. Benson was the first to describe certain physiological events as the *relaxation response*—a counterpoint to Hans Selye's notion of the *stress response*. Benson posited that during activities such as meditation, a person's heart-rate patterns, breathing rates, and hormone levels undergo changes that are beneficial to health. Trained as a cardiologist, he focused on the heart.

Like Selye's theories, those of Benson were popular with the lay public and with his patients but took decades to gain acceptance by the academic community. In the 1970s, long before such centers were in vogue, Benson established an institute of clinical mind-body medicine at Massachusetts General Hospital. Today it is called the Benson-Henry Institute for Mind Body

Medicine, and provides outpatient medical services, as well as training for healthcare professionals. The institute has a number of affiliates in locations across the United States, in Switzerland, and in Taiwan. One of its missions is to train healthcare professionals in a systematic, standardized way, to deliver mind-body interventions in conjunction with conventional Western medical therapies. To this end, Benson runs an annual continuing-education course at Harvard, which professionals from his affiliates and anyone else interested in these techniques can attend.

Both in developing a healthcare delivery program, and in pursuing communication with the lay public through his books and the media, Benson was ahead of his time. Like Selye, he at first alienated many of his academic colleagues, who frowned upon such mundane practices and viewed his studies on meditation and the relaxation response as "soft" science. A 1997 news article in *Science Magazine* described him this way: "Harvard Medical School cardiologist Herbert Benson has made a career out of pushing the biomedical research community to accept ideas once considered fringe. An early champion of the notion that stress can cause high blood pressure, he has promoted research on mind-body medicine for years—and earned a string of mainstream National Institutes of Health grants for his work."

Benson was by no means the only researcher who was studying meditation in the early 1970s, but he was the first to focus on the heart and to apply this technique to treating cardiovascular disease. Yet he didn't start out wanting to study meditation. Quite the opposite. In his clinical practice, he had noticed that patients' blood pressure increased during their regular checkups, so he decided to study the phenomenon. He performed studies on monkeys, training them to associate a reward (termination of a noxious stimulus) with elevated blood pressure. Just like Pavlov and his dogs, Benson was able to link the reward to a physiological response: an increase in blood pressure.

By the time Benson came on the scene, scientists had been studying meditation for more than three decades. One paper was published as early as 1937, a few came out in the 1940s and 1950s, and a great number appeared in the 1960s. Many of these studies reported on the effects of meditation on metabolism: oxygen consumption, body temperature, heart rate, and respiratory rate. But there were none on blood pressure. A researcher at UCLA, Robert Wallace, had published a landmark article in *Science* magazine showing that Transcendental Meditation (TM), as practiced by the Maharishi Mahesh Yogi, led to a hypometabolic state—something akin to hibernation, where heart and breathing rates slowed, and oxygen consumption and metabolism in the tissues decreased.

Though the paper was published in a highly respected academic journal, most mainstream researchers thought the topic still had a touchy-feely air. This was, after all, the Sixties, when techniques like meditation were beginning to sweep the country. Such practices conjured up a lifestyle that went counter to the prevailing power structure of academic medicine; they evoked long-haired, pot-smoking hippies who sang and danced on street corners wearing saffron robes and chanting phrases like "Hari Krishna." Even the name of the teacher, Maharishi Mahesh Yogi, who had developed a standardized method for TM that was taught across America, tended to evoke a cartoon character sitting atop a snowy peak and meditating in the lotus position. But Robert Wallace was from California, where such practices were embraced. Perhaps it was this attitude, and the availability of well-trained students of meditation provided by the Maharishi's schools in Los Angeles and Berkeley, which helped Wallace devise a rigorous technique for measuring the effects of meditation on metabolism—so rigorous that his work was accepted for publication in *Science*. Electrocardiograms, though taken on only five of the participants, showed that the technique could decrease heart rate by about five beats per minute.

Wallace was curious to know more. He had heard of Benson's work on blood pressure and wanted to know if the opposite could happen. Could his meditation techniques lower blood pressure, the way Benson's conditioning studies had elevated it? Benson was at first reluctant to collaborate, but eventually agreed, and he and Wallace designed a study that focused on the heart. It showed once again that this form of meditation lowered metabolic rate and decreased heart rate, though only by three beats per minute. The study was published the following year (1971) in the highly respected *Journal of Physiology*.

Not satisfied with observing the effects of a single episode of meditation on heart function, Benson went on to apply the technique over a twenty-five-week period, successfully treating patients with borderline high blood pressure. The method lowered blood pressure significantly: by seven to ten millimeters of mercury—a remarkable effect, given that no anti-hypertensive drugs were administered. Benson and Wallace were winning acceptance for the method by designing studies whose results were hard to refute. A fortuitous set of circumstances enabled Benson to take his physiological studies on meditation to the next level. He collaborated with Ary Goldberger to study the effects of different types of meditation breathing on heart-rate variability, an indication of the brain's stress or relaxation response.

It was Goldberger who approached Benson with a suggestion to collaborate, when he found out that the hospitals they worked at in Boston—Beth Israel and Deaconess—would be merging. He thought that a collaboration would help to cement the physical and administrative connection of these two institutions, and that the physical merger could thus have some positive spinoffs. He knew of Benson's studies on meditation, and thought it would be interesting to apply his physiological methods to studying the effects of Benson's techniques.

When I asked Goldberger why, besides that very practical reason, a skeptical scientist like him would want to study meditation, his immediate and emphatic response was: "I still am totally skeptical on everything. That is the scientific posture. I want to see the scientific data—actually what effect there is on the most unprocessed data you can have." He admitted, too, that he had become intrigued by meditation when learning about the Eastern tradition from a close collaborator, the statistical physicist Chung-Kang "C.K." Peng.

Yet it turned out there was another reason Goldberger had become interested in meditation, long before he met C.K. Peng or Herb Benson, and even before he went to medical school. The reason was his father, an internist and cardiologist. Goldberger recalled that his father "had a huge interest in psychosomatic medicine, even before it became mind-body medicine." About half of his father's library had "stuff related to EKG's and hard science," and the rest was devoted to psychosomatic medicine. "He must have had every book written about that field at the time." He was particularly interested in relaxation techniques, and taught these to his patients. "He talked about it all the time," and even taught the methods to his son. The talk and teaching and books had awakened young Goldberger's interest in the techniques. So when the two hospitals joined some twenty years later, Goldberger saw an opportunity to test the techniques in a rigorous, scientific way.

He and Benson teamed up to merge Goldberger's expertise in heart-rate variability methods and mathematical analysis with Benson's expertise in different forms of meditation and relaxation techniques. They decided to study breathing—the simplest element of these approaches that could be closely tied to rhythms of the heart. They chose eleven volunteers experienced in a form of Kundalini yoga that emphasizes coordination of breath, sound, movement, and attention. The participants had all practiced yoga at least five times per week for three to fifteen years. They were fitted with chest and abdominal bands that recorded breathing rate and depth, and heart monitors that continuously recorded heartbeats. They were then instructed to perform three types of breathing exercises. The first was relaxation-response breathing: they sat comfortably, allowing their breathing to become slow and easy. They were instructed to let their mind dwell on the mantra "Sat nam, whahe guru," and focus on it without effort as their breath went in and out. In the second exercise, they performed the so-called Breath of Fire, a smooth pattern of rapid breathing through the nose, powered by the diaphragm rather than the abdomen. The third and final exercise was bilateral segmented breathing, in which the breath is divided into eight equal steps on inhalation and eight on exhalation.

All of the participants reported feeling profoundly relaxed after the exercise, though the Breath of Fire is a much more energizing activity than the other two types. When Goldberger analyzed the heart-rate variability data, he was surprised to find that two of these forms of breathing meditation—the relaxation response and segmented breathing—were associated with an increase in heartbeat dynamics, rather than a quieting of the rhythm. In both types, breathing patterns became tightly yoked to heart rhythms at the same slow frequency. In the Breath of Fire, it was the opposite. There was an increase in heart rate and an uncoupling of breath rhythm from heart rhythm, suggesting an increase in the adrenalin component of the stress response.

The pattern observed in the relaxation response and segmented breathing has also been found in other forms of meditation, including Chinese Chi, yogic, and Zen traditions, and has even been found in people who pray with rosary beads.

Goldberger and Benson concluded that there are many paths to relaxation and that their effects on heart rhythms and breathing are complex; but attention to breathing seems to be an important component in all of these methods.

"I think of this as an unclenching," Goldberger says. "When the system gets overly tense, it is like a tight fist. It is locked. Somehow, by focusing your attention elsewhere, there is an unlocking, an unclenching of the fist. It is very striking." He describes the results with a note of awe in his voice: "There are big waves—the range of heart rate changes by thirty beats per minute. These are huge changes. The system is very plastic. This is exactly what you want. It is the opposite of a system locked to a characteristic frequency. It opens the state up." This is precisely what he said in his lectures on patterning: healthy heart rhythms produce the opposite of a straight line. Somehow, breathing types of meditation move the system from a rigid, nondynamic state to a plastic, healthy one.

Goldberger became so convinced that such methods could improve heart function that he collaborated in a study of the cardiac effects of Tai Chi, involving a group of patients with heart failure. The study showed that Tai Chi—another practice that combines slow purposeful movements, regular breathing, and meditation—can improve not only patients' subjective reports of quality of life, but can also enhance objective measures of cardiac function. From an outspoken skeptic, Goldberger became a firm proponent of Tai Chi as an intervention in heart disease.

Walking a labyrinth involves many of the features of Tai Chi: slow breathing, meditation, and gentle exercise. Though no one has tested this assumption, labyrinths might be another path to physiological relaxation through controlled breathing.

There are other kinds of walking meditations, practiced throughout the world. One involves use of the Buddhist prayer wheel—a large brass drum, often beautifully embellished with colorful symbols and geometrical designs. It is filled with tiny slips of paper on which prayers are written. The practitioner grasps a handle on its side and slowly walks around, turning the drum in the process. The pace is set by the weight of the heavy drum, which makes it impossible to go very fast. Breathing soon slows to a regular rate that matches the deliberate pace. Is there something about this leisurely form of exercise, besides the measured breathing, which blocks the stress response? Could it be the mild exercise, the walking, which is the source of the calming influence?

Many studies have shown that exercise improves mood. Low-grade exercise, like walking, produces results after just thirty minutes. Studies that compare exercise of various intensities show that low- to moderate-intensity exercise is most effective. This is the case for people who are healthy, for people who are ill with chronic pain or arthritis, for the elderly, and for people with depression. Not only do single bouts of exercise improve mood, but regular exercise can protect against depression. This may have something to do with the effects of exercise on nerve chemicals and brain hormones that are out of balance in depression. Regular exercise strengthens connections between nerve cells that produce the chemical serotonin, which is important in regulating mood. Nerve cells that produce the adrenalin-like nerve chemical norepinephrine become perturbed less easily. So exercise seems to have a beneficial effect, by improving nerve-cell connections that elevate mood and by decreasing connections that enhance the stress response. And all this, it turns out, is good for the immune system.

Moni Fleshner, a professor of physiology at the University of Colorado at Boulder, started her career as an exercise physiologist. An avid sports enthusiast, she was convinced that exercise was not only good for general health and mood, but could also affect immune function. With her long, straight blond hair and blue eyes, Fleshner could have succeeded equally well in the modeling profession, but she chose instead to pursue a topic that academics still considered fringe when she began to study it. With toughness, determination, and intelligence, she proved that exercise does in fact affect not only immune responses but also mood.

As a graduate student, Fleshner had noticed that when she exercised regularly, her mood improved and she was able to cope better with challenges. Also, some of her friends seemed more resilient and better able to cope than others. She wondered if exercise had anything to do with it.

Clinical literature published in the late 1980s and early 1990s showed that exercise could be used as an adjunct to treat depression. These studies had compared the efficacy of treating depression with serotonin re-uptake inhibitors (drugs like Prozac), alone or in combination with exercise, and found that when exercise was added to the treatment regimen, there were fewer relapses. The study that most impressed Fleshner—performed by Jonathan Brown and Judith Siegel and published in 1980—documented numbers of infectious illnesses during periods of low or high stress in teenage girls who were either sedentary or active. There was no difference between numbers of illnesses when the two groups of girls were not stressed. But during periods of high stress, the number of illnesses shot up in the sedentary girls and remained low in the active girls. Excited by these results, Fleshner designed a study looking at immunity in exercising rats. Her goal was to see if maintaining regular moderate levels of physical activity could change the way the body responds to immune challenges and stress.

Fleshner followed a well-established protocol that was known to produce cardiac fitness in rats. It was strikingly reminiscent of the exercise programs people follow at the gym after a sedentary period over the holidays. The rats went through an eight-week training program, running on a treadmill up a 10 percent grade five times per week. Treadmill velocity and running time were gradually increased in small increments to accommodate increases in the rats' fitness. The program included two five-minute warm-ups and one five-minute cool-down period. Increases in treadmill velocity and duration of run-time were implemented when the rats were able to maintain a level of exercise intensity for five consecutive days. At the end of the study, the rats' metabolism had increased, which was a good thing—but their immune responses were depressed, and there was evidence that their stress response was activated.

This result was unexpected. The findings looked more like a stress response than an indication of something that protected against stress. Others have obtained similar results, in rats and in people. A famous study of army rangers found that troops undergoing extremes of exercise succumbed more often to infectious illnesses, especially upper respiratory-tract infections. The doctors who studied these recruits found that their immune-cell function was depressed and stress hormones were elevated. The military decided to change the structure of the training so as to give the troops a rest in the middle of the period. Their immune systems were allowed to recover, and the soldiers were thus protected from infections during the last stages of training.

Fleshner modified the rats' exercise regime, making it less strenuous and less compulsory—allowing the rats to choose when they would jump on the running wheel, and letting them exercise over a period of four to six weeks. This program seemed to be less stressful and had more beneficial effects. Rats that engaged in regular moderate exercise showed an increase in several antibodies and immune cells important in the body's first line of defense against infection. They also made more antibodies when challenged with a vaccine. In other studies, Fleshner found an increase in brain chemicals that enhance moods and protect against depression—chemicals like dopamine and serotonin. She later collaborated with clinical researchers to show that regular moderate exercise has similar beneficial effects in people.

One question still bothered her: What was the source of these effects? Studies showed that adrenalin-like nerves and the chemicals they released in the spleen change the way immune cells behave in fighting infection. The work of two other women researchers, one in the United States and the other in the Netherlands, helped to solve the puzzle. Both started their careers when the field of psychoneuroimmunology, and certainly the professional societies that governed it, were dominated by men. Through their persistent, careful, and methodical research, the women managed not only to break new ground scientifically, but also, like Moni Fleshner, rose to the top of one of the major professional societies in their field.

An immunologist from Ohio State University, Virginia Sanders has spent her career studying the effects of adrenalin-like nerve chemicals on the activity of immune cells, especially the lymphocytes that produce antibodies to fight infection. She is a large, warm-hearted person who always seems to be enjoying her work tremendously and who acknowledges the importance of colleagues' support in her success, which has included election to the presidency of the PsychoNeuroImmunology Research Society. At an early stage, she was intrigued by a fact that had been known for decades: the spleen and other immune organs were laced with adrenalin-like nerves, which often touched the immune cells in these organs. Sanders wondered whether the nerve chemicals released by these nerves could have an effect on how immune cells functioned. It had been known since 1980 that the surface of immune cells contains receptor proteins which allow adrenalin-like nerve chemicals to bind to them—but no one knew what these receptors were doing there. Sanders demonstrated that adrenalin-like compounds can enhance some aspects of immune-cell activity, and suppress others.

Across the Atlantic, at the University of Leiden in the Netherlands, Cobi Heijnen (who also became president of the same research society), was studying immune cells called *T lymphocytes*. These cells are important in inflammation, and they make other immune cells grow and divide. They respond to bits of foreign material from the environment called antigens, and trigger the immune cascade. Furthermore, they hold the immune system's memory of such foreign material, so that each time you are exposed to the invader, your body can recognize it and quickly mount a response.

Heijnen, a tall woman with short curly blonde hair and a ready smile, often gives her lectures wearing jeans and stylish European-cut jackets. She began studying T lymphocytes in young patients with juvenile rheumatoid arthritis, which strikes before puberty. Clinicians had long known that if a patient with rheumatoid arthritis suffers a stroke, the arthritis disappears on the side of the body that is paralyzed. Heijnen wondered whether adrenalin-like nerves had anything to do with regulating the immune system and the course of arthritis. Like Sanders, she found that lymphocytes expressed receptors for adrenalin-like nerve chemicals on their surface, and also responded to adrenalin-like drugs.

Sanders and Heijnen showed that once adrenalin-like nerve chemicals attach to their receptors, they set off a whole series of events in immune cells that change the cells' function. In some cases the nerve chemicals enhance immune cells, and in other cases they depress them. What they do depends on dose. When you are exercising to the max, the overall effect of these hormones and nerve chemicals is to depress the cells' ability to fight infection. Something altogether different happens during milder exercise, such as walking.

When you walk at a regular pace, breathing deeply and evenly, the vagus nerve, with its soothing rhythms, takes over and overrides the adrenal gland, with its adrenalin and cortisol rush. The beating of your heart and the tempo of your breathing synchronize in calming, undulating waves. As you take a deep breath, your heart rate slows; as you let it out, your heart speeds up just a bit. The millisecond between beats increases and decreases in sync with these breaths. Your blood pressure falls; and instead of blood vessels clamping down to keep up blood flow to the vital organs, your heart pumps more strongly and effectively. The brake to your stress response has been engaged.

Moni Fleshner discovered that during strenuous exercise and at times of stress, the adrenalin-like nerves that permeate the spleen become depleted—they literally burn out. It is not the elevation in adrenalin in the blood that suppresses immune-cell activity during stress; rather, it is the depletion in the spleen that causes this, because a small amount of these adrenalin-like nerve chemicals is needed to help maintain immune-cell function. Regular moderate exercise prevents this depletion. As a result, there is less suppression of immune cells' ability to fight infection.

These findings have been borne out in people. Regular walking, just thirty minutes per day, bolsters the immune response, especially the cells that are the immediate defenders against infection. In elderly individuals who walk 3,000–10,000 steps per day, counted on a pedometer, it is the people who engage in moderate exercise (around 7,000 steps per day) whose immune systems show the strongest response. It is these walkers who have more first-line defense antibodies in their saliva—antibodies that are known to help prevent infections such as upper respiratory infections, colds, and sinusitis.

Together, these studies show that moderate exercise like walking, especially on a regular basis, not only enhances mood but also boosts the immune system. It could be that walking a labyrinth has many of these beneficial effects, though exactly which remains to be tested. No one has yet studied immune responses in people walking a labyrinth, but with new technologies, such research is now possible.

However it works, the labyrinth at Chartres has now been copied in thousands of places throughout North America, thanks to the initiative of Dr. Lauren Artess, canon pastor of Grace Cathedral in San Francisco. After a pilgrimage to Chartres, she hit upon the idea of copying its labyrinth onto a large portable canvas that can be rolled out anywhere. The design, forty-two feet in diameter, is usually printed full size on canvas and is rolled out on a regular basis in hospitals, clinics, and churches across America. Walking the labyrinth is becoming an accepted practice in complementary and alternative medicine.

When Ann Berger, the physician who directs the Pain and Palliative Care Unit at the National Institutes of Health (NIH) Clinical Center, decided that a labyrinth would be beneficial to her staff, her patients, and their families, she found it a bit trickier to implement than other mind-body interventions. But she was nothing if not persistent, and was committed to providing her staff and patients with every possible venue for improving their quality of life and reducing their stress.

Berger had originally trained as a nurse, obtaining her B.S. in nursing from New York University and a Master's in oncology nursing from the University of Pennsylvania. This training prepared her well for her eventual specialty in chronic-pain manage-

ment and palliative care—the clinical field that focuses on helping people heal, no matter how ill they are. Berger became
versed in the use of complementary and alternative mind-body
interventions to manage chronic pain and to improve quality of
life, techniques including meditation, massage, and acupunc-
ture. A survivor of breast cancer and open-heart surgery, she had
tried many of these herself and had even written a popular book
called *Healing Pain,* which discussed these approaches.

The old NIH Clinical Center, a federal hospital research facility, was built in 1953 as the nation's main hospital devoted entirely to clinical research. Patients with rare and difficult diseases
could come there to be treated free of charge with new experimental therapies; the results of these studies would advance scientific and medical knowledge and lead to new treatments. The
hospital was not devoted to primary, secondary, or even tertiary
care. Patients could not walk in off the street, and a doctor could
not send patients there to be treated unless they fit the criteria
of an ongoing research protocol addressing some aspect of their
illness.

In 2004, after years of construction, the new NIH Clinical
Center building was opened. It was connected to the old hospital through a series of bridges and corridors. Unlike the long,
barren, battleship-green hallways of the old "Building 10" (a
name perfectly suited to the sterility of its interior), the new hospital contains large, bright, airy spaces, including an enormous
seven-story atrium with a Zen-like pool in the middle of its pol-
ished granite floor, surrounded by chairs and café tables.

Berger's office in the Clinical Center is a wonder to behold. It
is filled with knick-knacks, mostly on a theme of tea: miniature
porcelain tea sets, odd porcelain cups, doll-sized teapots with
tiny tea parties sculpted on their covers, an inlaid Italian tea cart,
a floral-and-gold tea service, and every kind of tea imaginable.
When asked about this theme, Berger explains that these are for

her patients, their families, and the staff. Elaborate tea ceremonies, complete with hats and feather boas, are held for the patients and their families. Everyone gets to choose a favorite cup, hat, and boa, and they all have a grand time. "For us in palliative care," says Berger, "the patients and their family are really the unit of care."

At the NIH, Berger strove to provide her patients and staff with the best complementary and alternative interventions, to help improve their quality of life and reduce stress. Just before the Palliative Care Unit moved into the newly constructed Clinical Center, she and her staff found that finger labyrinths—miniature labyrinths in which you trace the path with your finger—helped to reduce stress. They routinely used these to alleviate not only their own stress, but also that of their patients. It was a way of relaxing by drawing the focus of attention away from the stressful situation.

Berger requested permission to install a full-size labyrinth in the Clinical Center. Although she had the blessing of the facility's director, others were not as supportive, perhaps because the device was unfamiliar and unproven—something that, in conventional Western medicine, was not based on evidence. But she succeeded in having one installed. When brochures announcing the labyrinth were printed and placed in the cafeteria, inviting staff to participate, she received angry phone calls from some scientists and physicians concerned about the appropriateness of putting a labyrinth in the Clinical Center. Was it safe? Was it effective? She assured them it could do no harm.

The labyrinth remains a very popular place for all who need respite from a hectic day. The healthcare staff use it just as much as the patients and their families, often visiting at lunchtime, to take a break from the pressures of their work.

The Clinical Center labyrinth is silk-screened on a large canvas. On the first and third Tuesday of every month, it is rolled out onto the floor of a wide atrium at the back of the hospital. To come upon this space, after navigating the warren of hospital corridors, is a surreal experience. The last place in the world one would expect to find a labyrinth is in the flagship hospital of one of the world's leading institutions in conventional medical research.

When you arrive, you are greeted by a friendly staff person who explains the principles of the labyrinth, the practicalities of taking off your shoes and donning paper booties, the importance of slow, quiet, deep breathing, and the need to take your time when walking along its path.

Standing at the entrance to the canvas labyrinth, you can see no route in or out—and if you try, you will defeat its purpose of putting you at ease. You should simply start. Step by step, follow the line that takes you to the center and then leads you back out to where you began. Trust that if you follow the path you will not get lost, and that you will come out feeling better than when you began. In many ways, this is a metaphor for any spiritual journey.

When you follow the path through a labyrinth, you have no need of landmarks. Yet elsewhere, these visual cues are crucial in helping you to navigate your environment: they tell you where you are going and where you have been. Two creative geniuses of the twentieth century, one an architect and the other a master of entertainment, applied to their work the essence of the way the brain uses landmarks in navigation, and the way these objects can trigger a full range of emotions. This synthesis forever changed the landscape of the built environment in which we live, to create spaces that can stimulate, excite, or calm. Who were these men and how did they accomplish this amazing feat? And can we learn from their experience to better design spaces that help us heal?

6

FINDING YOUR WAY . . .

In 2006, the Society for Neuroscience invited Frank Gehry to deliver the keynote address at its annual meeting in Atlanta. The lecture one was of a series entitled "Dialogues between Neuroscience and Society"—and by that time, the members of the organization, and neuroscientists in general, were feeling more comfortable with the idea of sponsoring a major lecture on a topic outside their field. The previous year's lecture, by the Dalai Lama, had broken new ground, convincing the audience of pure scientists that it was important to think about how their research affected society, and how, in turn, crucial questions beyond the realm of science influenced their work.

According to *AIArchitect*, the newsletter of the American Institute of Architects, "Gehry's presentation drew an estimated crowd of 7,000. 'For a non-scientist to attract that many people speaks to the success of Gehry's lecture,' Society for Neuroscience President Stephen Heinemann said. 'This is an experimental series looking at the top creative people in their field. We want to look at the best and get a feel for what our minds can do.'"

Gehry described his creative process. His talk was peppered with endearing, self-deprecating, Woody Allen–type humor that revealed the vulnerability of a creative genius who, while pushing the envelope and opening up new worlds, had to overcome fear and anxiety. It was this aspect of his remarks that resonated with the audience, especially the younger scientists, who themselves were attempting, with some uncertainty, to test the boundaries of the possible.

Gehry turns architecture on its head by designing buildings that don't even look like buildings. Instead of neat, square boxes, his structures are fluid, crumpled, metal-clad forms—eccentric, eye-catching landmarks. Viewed from afar, these unique shapes stand out from the rest of the buildings in any skyline. But if an entire city were made up of Gehry buildings, they would no longer be landmarks. It is their differentness that makes them stand out in a cityscape—a differentness that is at once exciting and anxiety-provoking and, as a result, memorable. These qualities are the characteristics of a landmark. Gehry did not start from principles of neuroscience, but intuitively tapped into an essential element of how the brain works. He knew how to create features that maximize the brain's ability to recognize, respond to, and remember differentness.

According to popular myth, his design process includes crumpling up a sheet of paper and studying its folds. Gehry himself says that he starts with lots of scribbles and hands these to his young assistants, who somehow understand what he is trying to say and translate them into the fluid shapes that become his buildings. In fact, the process is quite rigorous and involves a great many iterations. The final form is based not only on the initial, often organic inspiration—a fish, a horse's head, a sail—but also on the building's eventual occupants, its intended use, the configuration of the site, and the neighboring structures.

The original inspirations for Gehry's Guggenheim Museum in Bilbao, Spain, were stone sculptures by French medieval and Renaissance artists and the ancient statues of Greece and Rome. It was their draperies that inspired him, their folds that convey the warmth and suppleness of fabric. But rather than making his folds out of stone, Gehry made them of titanium, and used this metal to clothe his building in a lustrous skin. His hunch was that the look of soft folds of fabric would evoke positive emotions in the viewer, emotions arising from childhood associations with mothers' skirts and comforting blankets.

Gehry's buildings are visually striking from afar and help you to orient yourself in a city. Drive down Interstate 101 and exit in downtown Los Angeles, and you come to a spaghetti mix of access ramps and poorly labeled one-way streets. Your anxiety peaks as you try to avoid accidentally getting back on the freeway. But if you catch sight of the shiny façade of the Gehry-designed Walt Disney Concert Hall, you know exactly where you are and your anxiety diminishes.

Up close, his buildings cause a different sort of emotional flip. They nudge you toward anxiety, until you enter them. From the outside, all that's visible is a disjointed structure of searing, blinding-shiny metal and glass. You might expect that the inside would be equally jarring, perhaps made of the same sharp, hard, industrial materials. But walk into the Disney Concert Hall and you immediately feel a sense of calm. The interior is both cool and warm. Entering from the ticket office, you encounter an angular tree-like structure rising to the ceiling, its trunk and branches clad in pale yellowish Douglas fir. As your eyes become accustomed to the indoor light, you realize you're in a forest of these "trees"—cleverly disguised support columns and ventilation ducts. Even the soaring ceiling and walls are made of wood. All of the lines are curves, reminiscent of waves—water waves, sound waves. Portions of the travertine floors are covered with brownish-yellow carpeting, mottled with images suggesting multicolored roses. The overall effect is of a stylized woodland.

At every turn, you confront this juxtaposition of shapes and colors that recall nature but make no attempt at mimicry. And at every turn, you glimpse the outside world. You can't help wondering: How did Gehry do this? From the outside, the building appears to have no windows, no views of the outdoors. Disconcerted, you suspect it's as dark as a mausoleum inside. But in fact every space in the building, including the concert hall, affords a view of the outside world through glass skylights and pierced walls.

During a panel discussion at the Society for Neuroscience meeting, I asked Gehry about the tension between novelty and familiarity in his buildings. I observed that they can be reassuring landmarks, yet also generate stress because they are so unconventional, and I wondered whether he incorporated any design features to manage that potential stress reaction. Gehry said he was aware that when viewed up close, his buildings might cause anxiety because they don't conform to people's expectations of how a building should look. For this reason, he includes elements that he calls "handrails"—features that allow people to orient themselves with respect to calming, exterior views or stabilizing points of reference within the building. He hit upon this device entirely by instinct. Such design elements enabled him to minimize the anxiety generated by his buildings, and to move viewers' responses from the zone of discomfort to the zone of excitement.

As much as Gehry has wanted to jar people and cities out of their complacency, another great creative genius of the twentieth century and the namesake of his concert hall, Walt Disney, wanted to do the opposite: smooth out all of the warts and wrinkles and grime in the landscape and make people feel completely at ease. Gehry designed the building for Disney's widow, Lillian. Although some think it looks like a rose ("a rose for Lilly"), Gehry says what he really had in mind were "two sails with the wind behind you." The project took a decade, slowed by funding shortages, design alterations, earthquakes, and the 9/11 terrorist attacks. The hall finally opened in 2003.

Though their creative works seem to have little in common,

Disney and Gehry shared important character traits. Lillian once said to Gehry that had her husband lived twenty years longer, she was sure they would have become fast friends. Both held to concepts of design that not only captured the spirit of their times, but broke all existing rules. Both worked tirelessly to turn their vision into reality, in the face of much opposition and stiff odds. Both combined artistic genius with the latest technological advances and materials available to them. Gehry and Disney were also kindred spirits in the way they created and employed landmarks to orient and guide. And both used elements of surprise to excite and inspire, while counterbalancing these with familiar features to reassure their audiences.

When Walt Disney came up with the idea of bringing the audience into his movies—instead of just letting viewers sit in a dark space and watch images on a screen—he chose twelve of his most talented animators to help him do this. He called them "Imagineers." When you enter a Disney theme park, you're crossing a threshold into an imaginary world that was created, down to its minutest detail, to fool your brain into thinking it is real. Disney's team played on many aspects of perception and behavior, and turned them to its advantage. The results are so lifelike and enticing, that close to forty million adults and children visit Disneyland, Walt Disney World, and Epcot every year.

John Hench was one of the original dozen Imagineers who created Disneyland in Anaheim, California, and Disney World in Orlando, Florida (opened in 1955 and 1971, respectively). The parks were designed to take people from fear and anxiety to hope and relief. How did the Imagineers accomplish this? Hench was not only a brilliant artist and engineer, but also a voracious reader. He subscribed to more than a hundred magazines and journals of all types, including periodicals on psychology and human behavior. He was a student of Freud and Jung and was fascinated by the psychology of perception, in those days an emerging field. Relatively little was known about the neuroscience of perception, and the only way to learn this was to work it out by trial and error—which he did. Over the years, he learned precisely how much visual data and how much perceptual time viewers needed, in order to be convinced that an image was real.

When Disney proposed to his animators that they create mood-altering spaces that people could enter and that could give the illusion of distance, height, and speed, he was asking his artists to take their knowledge of cinematography and animation to a whole new level. Fortunately, at the same time that the Disney Studios were developing animation, they were also making forays into movies and television and were employing designers to create three-dimensional sets. It was also becoming possible to build life-size, three-dimensional, moving figures: robots. So the animators had the technical tools, plus knowledge about illusion and perception, with which to create fantasy spaces that simulated reality.

What is it about Disneyland rides like "Pirates of the Caribbean" that makes you believe you're entering a pirates' cave in the Caribbean and not a warehouse on a lot in California or Florida? What is it that makes you believe that pieces of brown and gray spray-painted cardboard are rocks in the cave? There is one thing that has to happen before anything else—an age-old theatrical trick: the lights go out. It gets dark.

Once all visual cues have been removed via this simple method, the animators can gradually add back whatever cues they like, to create a new world for you. In "Pirates of the Caribbean," you start from the sunny grounds of a New Orleans mansion and walk up a sloping brick ramp that brings you into a genteel southern home. Gradually the ramp turns into wooden planks; you can feel them under your feet. The scene shifts to a fishing wharf. The light grows dimmer. The sounds change from those of a harborside restaurant—music, the clatter of cutlery and plates, the voices of diners—to those of the Bayou and the swamp: crickets and lapping water. You step into a boat bobbing on a murky lagoon. Now only lanterns light your way.

As the boat glides forward, you leave behind the tempting smells of Cajun cooking and pick up the musty, earthy scent of the pirates' cave. You hear a tune familiar to most Americans— "Oh, Susanna!" (sung a bit off key)—and see a banjo player singing and strumming in a rocking chair. Then something unexpected happens: the boat abruptly drops down a steep incline as it enters the cave. When you walked up the ramp to enter the ride, leaving the sunlight behind, you didn't realize you were rising an entire story above the ground. The drop completes your separation from the familiar world outside and sets the mood—fear and anxiety—for the rest of the ride. Perhaps without realizing it, Disney's Imagineers have used one of the most powerful triggers of the brain's stress response to set it off— namely a sudden, unexpected change. All those brain hormones and nerve chemicals that make you feel stressed and anxious have been let loose. You now know viscerally as well as visually that you have entered a new world and should expect the unexpected.

John Hench, who designed the "Pirates of the Caribbean" ride, also knew that there was more to perception than just the mechanics of the sensory organs. He knew about Jungian psychology and classical mythology. He knew that people carry with them deep associations born of universal stories and ancient myths. We may not be aware of these associations and often don't know where they come from, but they can color our reactions to a place or an image or a story. When we experience our environment, we not only perceive the physical elements in it, but we also try to make sense of the story it tells. When we enter a new space, we look for logical patterns and connections. If we can't find any, we feel unsettled.

Just before the boat drops, you notice a powerful image at the cave's entrance: a skull and crossbones, symbol of pirates and death. John Hench brilliantly coupled these mythic associations with physical cues employing tricks of lighting, sound, and movement, in order to maximize people's apprehension. According to a former Imagineer who worked with Hench, he also believed that at some level visitors would know they were entering a Freudian world of dreams—the realm of the unconscious. He knew that people who came to Disney's theme parks were seeking an adrenalin rush—the heightened sense of aliveness that comes with danger—yet at the same time wanted to feel safe, comfortable, and in control. His rides delivered. They created simulated threats that people could manage. Hench understood a fundamental truth: that imagined stress can be as powerful a trigger of the stress response as a real threat, and that the more control you have over that threat, the less stressed and the more stimulated you feel.

Indeed, when you enter a Disney theme park, you experience a blend of comfort and excitement. One of its main attractions is that it offers you Main Street America—a nostalgic America that existed in some imaginary past. This is not the Main Street America in which you grew up. But it's the Main Street where you would *like* to have grown up—a secure place filled with happy people, happy buildings, happy smells. It's the street that existed in Disney's memory of the town where he grew up— Marceline, Missouri, just outside Kansas City.

The Main Streets of Disneyland and Disney World do not actually resemble the main street of Marceline, as it was when Disney's family lived there (1906–1911). Disney was only nine when they moved away, but those five years left an indelible mark on him. His theme park Main Streets reflect what he saw in his mind's eye, when he went back to Marceline in his memory. Photos from the era show that the real Marceline was a dusty place whose main street was a windswept dirt road lined with two-story brick buildings. The awnings were drab, certainly not the gaily colored ones of Disneyland's Main Street. The town-scape was punctuated by crooked telegraph poles, not romantic lampposts. There was no Cinderella Castle in the distance, just the flat, flat, Missouri-Kansas horizon.

Disney re-created not the actual place, but the emotional ex-periences he had there—the sense of hope and freedom and bright expectation that animate a happy childhood. So success-ful was Disney in letting us into his emotional memory, that sim-ply by buying a ticket and walking into the park, we can share the emotions that he experienced in childhood and that stayed with him throughout his life. So successful was he in designing space and place to evoke an emotion and make you act in a cer-tain way, that his principles of design have been incorporated into virtually every public space in America.

If all you felt when you entered a Disney theme park were comfort, you would get bored and quickly leave. Disney couldn't force you to stay, so he had to find a way to make you move into and through the park. To do this, he inserted what he called "wienies" throughout. These were landmarks that stood out from the rest of the park and enticed people to move toward them, just as a wienie—a hot dog, a wiener—entices people to reach for it at a ballpark.

We know from the study of human movement that the brain searches for and identifies landmarks as we move, and that land-marks are very important in our memories of place and space. So a strategically located landmark is sure to make a person move toward it. In order to be a landmark, an object must have several characteristics. It needs to be big enough to be seen from a dis-tance. It needs to be different from its surroundings, so that it stands out, the way Gehry's buildings do. It needs to evoke some positive associations in order to draw you toward it. And it needs to be memorable. Disney knew all this intuitively and from experience. During World War I, he had spent a lot of time in Europe as an ambulance driver, and he returned there many times. He was fascinated by the old towns, where winding streets often led to a castle on a hill. He and his designers knew that castles are romantic, that they exert a magnetic attraction, and that they are universally associated with fairy tales. So he put a castle at the end of Main Street.

When you enter Disneyland, you do not at first see the Castle. You walk into a large open space—the Town Square. A band is playing on the green; an American flag is being raised or lowered to the tune of the national anthem. There's a firehouse to your left and charming old houses on every side. You stop and take in the scene, gradually leaving the real world behind. Your mood begins to change and you relax. You become a character on Disney's stage.

Then you notice a street leading out of the square, away from the main entrance gate. And the moment you round the corner, you see the Castle: a pinkish-gray turreted wonder straight out of *Cinderella* or *Sleeping Beauty*. It's at the far end of Main Street. But as you walk toward it, you're distracted by the street's tempting stores, which have old-fashioned façades and are filled with toys, pretty hats, ice cream, candies, and fudge. You can even smell the fudge as you walk past, because the Imagineers hit upon the idea of venting the cooking exhaust toward the street—a trick now used by restaurants all over the world to attract customers inside. More fudge is sold today on Disney's Main Street than almost anywhere else in America. Why? Because we have learned to associate the smell of fudge with comfort and home and childhood. You cannot resist stopping, gazing at the shopwindows, and walking through the door. And once inside, you buy the fudge.

Then you remember the Castle and continue on your way. But the landscape changes again. The street widens and you're presented with more wienies: thatched-roof buildings, a large mountain, an immense futuristic structure. Now you must decide where you want to go. You're standing in another large square, this one provided with benches, popcorn carts, and ice cream vendors. These cues tell you that there's no hurry about making your decision—you can take the time to enjoy a snack. Here is where you see visitors huddled in family groups, children tugging at their parents' elbows and pointing to where they want to go, adults poring over maps and guidebooks, until a decision is reached and they head off to explore another attraction.

When you move toward your next landmark, you pass through what the Imagineers call a "cross-dissolve." In filmmaking, this refers to a technique in which one scene slowly melts into the following one. In Disney's parks, each space slowly dissolves into the next as visitors walk along, so that they gradually become aware of having left one world and arrived at another. The Imagineers accomplished this by adding cues, perceived through all the senses, which signal the new land you are approaching, and at the same time subtracting cues from the one you've left behind. This was done so cleverly that you're not even aware your surroundings have changed until you get to your destination. As you move, say, from the plaza at the end of Main Street into Adventureland, the concrete pavement turns to gravel beneath your feet; the melodies of music grinders and ice cream trucks give way to the sounds of jungle creatures; the scent of popcorn is replaced by that of exotic spices; the architecture shifts from early twentieth-century America to an amalgam of desert-oasis bazaar and thatched-roof tropical structures.

Disney and his Imagineers have worked out a way to guide your behavior. They take advantage of the way your brain absorbs sensory clues about its environment, and use landmarks to make you walk in a certain direction: toward the Castle. With enticing aromas, colored baubles, and cheerful music, they induce you to slow down along Main Street and stop at the hub where the full range of possible adventures is presented to you. They skillfully change your mood—making you feel comfortable and at home in a charming, safe, imaginary past, then anxious and frightened, then safe again. They succeed in pacing your movements through the park in a measured way. And they do all this without saying a word.

As you navigate these places, your brain is constantly receiving myriad inputs: visual cues that tell you where you are heading, and internal cues that tell you where you have been. Different animals rely on each of these navigation methods to various degrees. Bumblebees use primarily visual cues—the angle of the sun and patterns in the sky—to navigate their "bee-lines." Spiders rely more on internal cues from strain-sensing receptors on their legs. Mammals use a combination of both types of information.

The internal cues, known collectively as *proprioception,* include sensations from your inner ear (your balance system) and from your muscles and joints—sensations that tell you how far you've traveled. It's as if the brain had its own pedometer, so that even if you are blindfolded you can generally find your way back to where you started. This is how blind persons find their way and how pilots in the early days of aviation navigated, "by the seat of their pants."

It's the combination of proprioceptive and visual cues that ensure the success of another Disneyland ride, "Soarin' over

California," which makes you feel as if you're flying even though you're only a few feet off the floor. When you "lift off," you feel the seat vibrating under you and the chair tilts backward. Your feet dangle as the seat swings gently back and forth. These sensations and the breeze blowing past your face create the illusion that you're in a glider. But you also have a panoramic view projected on the bowl-shaped movie screen all around you, and this makes the ride amazingly real. The angle of the seat and the bumpiness of the vibrations are perfectly coordinated with the visuals as you suddenly burst through the clouds, swoop down over the Golden Gate Bridge, and skim over rivers, beaches, and mountaintops. If not for the visual cues, you'd merely feel that you were in a vibrating, tilting chair, instead of soaring over California. If the proprioceptive cues didn't exactly match the visual cues, the experience would seem less realistic and you might get motion sickness. Besides telling your brain that you're moving when in fact you are not, the breeze blowing past your face also helps ward off queasiness.

When you navigate a path, such as Main Street in Disneyland, you need both visual and proprioceptive cues to find your way and to remember where you are going. Deprived of visual cues, sighted people make errors when navigating but can still get to their goal by using proprioception. Hence the fun of games like Pin the Tail on the Donkey, which would be less entertaining if there weren't a distinct possibility of getting it right. To compensate for lack of sight, blind people learn to be very sensitive to internal and nonvisual cues, including proprioception, sound, and smell.

As you walk, you perceive objects in a sequence and form sequential memories of what you see. Your proprioceptive system also registers segments of the path in sequence. When remembering place, you can play back your visual recollections in random order. It is the proprioceptive cues—which depend on your moving within that space rather than just looking at it—that need to be replayed in the correct sequence in order for you to remember them well. The process can be compared to driving yourself around a new city, as opposed to being driven as a passenger. A driver remembers a route after just a few tries, much faster and much better than when just viewing it from the passenger seat.

There's an entire field of architecture devoted to navigation. It's called *way-finding*. Architects know that people have two ways of navigating: one using landmarks and the other using grids. Cities usually conform to one pattern or the other. Rome and Paris are fine examples of landmark cities; Manhattan is a grid. When finding your way around Rome, you move from one landmark to another—meandering through winding streets that often change their name and make the whole process quite confusing. Try to go from the Spanish Steps to the Colosseum, and you're likely to circle around to where you started unless you keep searching for landmarks along the way—famous fountains, the Capitol, the Forum. In the ancient quarters of Paris, buildings block the sunlight from the crooked, narrow streets—the Rue de Chasse Midi literally means "the street that chases away the noon." But fix your gaze on landmarks like Sacré Coeur, the Tour Eiffel, the Tour St. Jacques, or Notre Dame Cathedral, and you can quickly find your way. This perhaps explains the popularity of tourist guidebooks that show aerial views of streets and 3-D drawings of landmarks and buildings to help you get your bearings.

In Manhattan it is much simpler. Walk west on 42nd Street to Broadway and you find Times Square. Walk south on 5th Avenue to 34th Street and you come to the Empire State Building. This is a landmark recognized around the world, but when you are walking around New York, you needn't look up to find your way to it. You need only count your steps and the numbers of streets you've crossed.

Most of us use both ways to navigate—landmarks and grids— but some of us are better at one than the other. Women tend to navigate using landmarks, and men tend to use grids. This can be exasperating when you're getting directions from someone whose skills are the opposite of yours. If you're a landmark person, and are told to go half a mile north on Main Street, then turn left on Oak and go thirty yards west, this may drive you into a frenzy. But if you're a grid person, and are told to drive a few blocks on Main until you get to a fast food restaurant, then turn left and drive a while until you see the firehouse, this may drive you equally berserk.

A rat in a water maze routinely uses landmarks to navigate. Rats love to swim—especially the brown Norway rat that came to America from Europe in the holds of ships three or four hundred years ago. Put a rat in a small plastic pool (used in laboratories, resembling a wading pool) and it will immediately jump into the water and swim. If there is a platform in the middle, just below the surface, it will quickly learn to head for that. On the first try, it will need a bit of time to find the platform, but after several tries it learns the way. Yet it needs to see the platform in the water in order to orient itself and get there. Now make the water opaque by adding a little milk. If the rat can't see the platform, it will become confused and anxious and will swim around until it eventually finds it. But put some visual cues on the wall around the pool—simple shapes of different colors (a big red triangle on one wall, a blue square on another)—and the rat will quickly learn to fix its sights on these landmarks. Curtains, patterns on the wall, and pieces of equipment will work too. After a couple of tries, the rat easily learns to find its way to the platform. This test, called the *Morris water maze,* is a standard way to test the effects of all sorts of environmental factors on learning and memory.

Matt Wilson, a scientist at MIT, often lectures on the neuroscience of navigation. He does a hilarious rendition of the abrupt head movements of a rat as it searches through a maze. Looking like a cartoon character that stepped out of an Egyptian tomb drawing, Wilson turns his head one way, straight black hair whipping his cheek, and moves one leg forward. Then he turns his head in the opposite direction and moves the other leg. The gestures illustrate how closely head movement is linked to spatial navigation.

There are two very important groups of nerve cells that form a network crucial to navigation through space. They're located in and near the hippocampus—the structure that reminded early anatomists of a seahorse. One set of nerve cells determines your position in space, and the other set responds to head direction. One forms an internal map, the other an internal compass.

Not surprisingly, the nerve cells that register location in space are called *place cells.* In his studies on rats, Wilson surgically implants an electrode in the hippocampus and measures the electrical firing of single nerve cells. While the rat is under anesthesia, a small metal helmet, marked in millimeters in three planes, is placed on its head and coordinates are fixed so that the electrode can be angled into place. When the rat wakes up from surgery, it goes about its day quite normally, with its tiny electrode-crown, ready to be attached to a recording instrument. When the electrode linked to the place region of the brain is hooked up to a computer, you can watch different cells light up on the screen with electrical impulses as the rat moves through various spaces. If the rat is moving through a maze shaped like a plus sign, you can see waves of nerve cells become active in the shape of a plus sign. These cells tell the rat exactly where it is at any particular moment. The same is true for humans: the part of the brain that guides our path carries a constantly shifting map of our surroundings.

It turns out that place cells perform another very important function: they pull together all the sensory inputs we receive, a process necessary for the creation of an integral sense of place. In Disney's theme parks, as you move through a cross-dissolve, you are receiving inputs from your senses of vision, hearing, smell, and touch. You integrate these cues into a whole, and it is the combination that tells you where you are. Every particular place you have experienced has an overall feel which is different from that of any other place. How do all those sensory cues form a map and give you that sense of place? How do they get stuck together?

The problem of sensory binding has been difficult for neuroscientists to solve. When it comes to spatial integration, hippocampal place cells seem to be the key. Each place cell receives inputs from many sources, including internal proprioceptive cues, visual cues, and other sensory cues like smell and touch and hearing. Visual cues are the strongest when you're navigating; next come smells and then motion cues, in order of importance. The hippocampus and its place cells, then, are both the integrator and the mapmaker in your brain. Integration involves other parts of the brain, including the parietal lobe and some parts of the cortex, but hippocampal place cells play a leading role. By constantly uploading many different kinds of sensory signals and outputting a single stream of electrical signals, they are responsible for assembling all the bits and creating a multidimensional, multisensory image of where you are in space.

There is another essential ingredient in the formation of an image of place, and this ingredient is memory. When moving through a cross-dissolve, you are forming sequential memories of what you see and what you feel as you navigate toward each landmark. If you couldn't remember all of those sensations and locations, you wouldn't know where you came from or where you were heading. Memory is every bit as crucial to our understanding of place as direct experience. There are many things we remember about a place and many different kinds of memory processes that help us to integrate bits and pieces of the outside world into specific images within our head—places we carry around with us wherever we go.

One way researchers have teased apart all the different brain regions involved in memory is by studying people who have sustained brain damage resulting in very specific kinds of memory loss. These patients' deficits shed light on how memory works in all of us. It's like trying to figure out why a ceiling light doesn't work—the problem could be in the bulb, the switch, or the wiring in between. Checking and replacing each part of the circuit will tell you how that circuit was set up in the first place. One woman did more than anyone else to work out the circuits of memory, in a remarkable fiifty-year collaboration with a patient whose memory was impaired.

7

. . . AND LOSING IT

At 3:00 A.M. one night in 1953, psychologist Brenda Milner arrived in Hartford, Connecticut, by train from Montreal, Canada, to examine a patient with severe memory loss: H.M. This was to become a decades-long collaboration between psychologist and patient which would shed light on the very nature of how memory works.

In the early 1950s, Wilder Penfield, a neurosurgeon who had established McGill University's Montreal Neurological Institute, had developed a method for removing the diseased part of the brain where seizures originated. Penfield had hired the young Brenda Milner, from Cambridge, England, and tasked her with determining, before the surgery, where the seizures were coming from. Sophisticated imaging technologies were then still decades in the future, and all Milner had at her disposal were psychological tests. But she and Penfield had perfected a technique that enabled them to map what different parts of the brain do.

Penfield was always conservative, removing as little of the brain as possible at first, so that some patients had to return for a second operation before their seizures were quelled. One such patient, P.B., a forty-six-year-old engineer, had returned for surgery after only a small portion of his temporal lobe had been removed. Milner's testing after the first operation showed that all of P.B.'s mental functions were intact. But his seizures persisted, and on the second operation Penfield removed a bit more of the temporal lobe, including the hippocampus. When P.B. awoke from the surgery, he suddenly said—rather sarcastically, according to Milner—"What have you people done to my memory?" Milner tested him again, and sure enough, although his immediate recall was unimpaired, his recent memory was gone. He could not remember when his wife had visited or who Milner was. This suggested that the hippocampus had something to do with the formation of new memories.

At first, Milner and Penfield thought this result might be unique to P.B. But when they saw a similar case a year later, they knew they were onto something of broader significance. They reported the two cases at a national meeting and began to search for other patients, in an effort to understand the cause. That's when they got a call from Dr. William Beecher Scoville in Hartford, saying that his patient H.M. might have a similar problem.

In 1953, H.M. was twenty-six years old and had severe intractable epilepsy. Scoville, who had been following Penfield's technique, went one better: he removed the deep part of both temporal lobes and most of the hippocampus. Immediately after he performed this surgery two things happened: H.M.'s seizures decreased dramatically, to only two per year, and he developed permanent severe amnesia. His recollection of events prior to the surgery was normal, but his memory loss going forward was virtually complete. He could not remember anything new, regardless of the type of memory he was asked to recall (events, people, faces, general knowledge, music, numbers, mazes) and regardless of the type of sensory stimulus that was used to jog his memory (visual, auditory, smell, or touch). He could not create new memories, though he had some limited recollection of events and people he had encountered before his surgery, including his mother, his father, and his surgeon.

Yet H.M. retained one surprising part of his memory. Though he could not find his way around a maze, he was able, at Milner's urging, to draw an accurate representation of the floor plan of a house that he moved into five years after his surgery and that he lived in for sixteen years. He did this on two occasions: eight years after moving in, and three years after moving out to another house.

This type of memory is called *topographic memory*. The fact that H.M. was able to accomplish this mapping task shows that other brain areas in the temporal lobes, in addition to the hippocampus, are important in this type of memory.

In 2008, at the age of ninety, Milner described her landmark experiments in a keynote lecture at a meeting of the Society for Neuroscience. She received a standing ovation from the more than four thousand neuroscientists in the audience. A tiny, energetic woman who retains a slight British accent, Milner still goes to work every day and continues to publish her research. She delivered her fast-paced lecture with grace and humor—without the aid of notes—and used vivid anecdotes to bring her patients to life. After the ovation, she was surrounded at the podium by a crowd of admiring colleagues and students, many of whom were young enough to be her great-grandchildren. They brandished digital cameras and held up cell phones to snap pictures of their idol—a rock star of neuroscience.

Brenda Milner's studies of H.M. have become classics in the field. They have shed light on how the brain makes memories and what parts of the brain govern each part of memory, including how we remember space and place.

There is no single region where memories are preserved in your brain. The brain is not a keepsake box into which you drop a thing to be remembered, and then open it up again when you need to take it out. Memory is a continuous process with many parts. There are various places in the brain where memories are created, then cemented, then retrieved. Different regions of the brain are involved in remembering different kinds of things. Memory of place and space mostly occurs in the hippocampus and a collection of adjacent structures, including the amygdala (the brain's fear center). These make up the *hippocampal complex,* a structure that is also very important in the recollection of biographical episodes, the events that happen to you. This type of memory is called *episodic memory.* Memory of general knowledge and facts (such as the famous names and faces you learn in history class) is called *semantic memory* and is controlled by other parts of the brain, though the hippocampus may be involved as well. The things you do and the order in which you do them are remembered in still another region, a network of brain areas that include the *striatum.* The process through which you acquire such memories is called *procedural memory* or *habit formation.* This involves the same kind of learning that Pavlov used to train his dogs—conditioning—but in this case you learn to associate various parts of a task, such as a movement with a visual cue. Learning to type without looking at the keyboard, or to play the piano by sight-reading, or even to walk or swim, are memories in this category.

Memories can also be divided into different types according to whether or not you are aware of them. *Declarative* or *explicit* memory is the kind in which you consciously recall facts and events; *nondeclarative* or *implicit* memory is the unconscious awareness of features you have previously learned about a thing. If someone shows you a glass bowl, you know that it is heavy and that if you drop it, it will break. If you see a feather, you know that it is light and that it will float gently to the ground when dropped. Those are implicit memories.

There is also a certain pace to the formation of a memory. The first part happens very fast—in the range of a few thousandths of a second to a few minutes. Fully cementing a memory, so that it lasts for years and years, may take days or weeks of repetition and requires the nerve cells to produce proteins and grow new connections. The more time that elapses from the formation of a memory to the time you retrieve it, the more vague and blurry it gets. There are several theories as to why this happens and what parts of the brain are involved in recent versus remote memories, particularly memories of place.

Some researchers believe there is a map of your environment inside your head, mostly in the hippocampal complex. This creates a spatial image in which events that you experience are embedded. Others suggest that recent memories are housed in the hippocampus, while older ones are archived in other parts of the brain. A third theory incorporates parts of these two; it proposes that autobiographical episodes are held in the hippocampal complex, but that each time a memory is retrieved, a new memory trace is formed. Each memory would then have many traces, which are held in various places in the brain. The complete explanation has yet to be worked out. What we do know is that when the hippocampus is involved, a memory is particularly vivid, especially with respect to the place where it was formed. It also has emotional qualities and personal significance.

Think of an early childhood memory. If it's an event, you'll probably think of it in the context of a place. You will be able to visualize the arrangement of the furniture in the living room, the location of the television set, and where the coffee table was when you fell against its sharp edge and cut your chin. In this case, the memory of the event is intimately connected to the memory of the place. It is also connected to the memory of the emotion you felt when you hurt yourself. Your hippocampal complex has become activated and is doing this work for you.

Memory not only is important in defining the shape of the place you're in, but also tells you something about the purpose of that place. Think of what you do when you wake up in the morning. You get out of bed and head for the bathroom. You know this room is a bathroom, and that the room you just left is a bedroom, because there are certain objects in each that tell you what the room is for. There is a sink and a toilet and a bathtub in one, and a bed and dresser in the other. Though you're unaware of it, these cues tell you not only what the places are, but what you should do in them. You know that you should not sleep in the bathtub or bathe in the bed. This is the same kind of memory that helps you to construct and decipher scenes made up of the objects you see.

Besides knowing what each room does, you also know how to get from one to the other. You know how to get from the bed to the bathroom, even with your eyes closed, or in the pitch dark. This is something you have learned by repetition, and the route is stored in your memory. But wake up in a hotel room and you may stumble into a wall or stub your toe on a chair before reaching the bathroom.

Memory of events and places is also crucial to our sense of self. Although many brain regions contribute to our sense of identity—including the parts that govern conscious will, feelings of love and affiliation, and beliefs and desires—the hippocampus and the memories it encodes play a very important part. They form an ever-changing image of ourselves in the context of our world.

All of your childhood memories, all of the memories you acquire every day of your life—what you have done, where you have done it, and how you felt while doing it—get stuck together. The collection in its entirety tells you who you are. If your memories start to fade, so do your sense of place and your sense of self. Start losing them and you lose a little bit of yourself with each memory that disappears.

Now imagine you have an illness that impairs your memory—an illness like Alzheimer's disease that leaves long-term memory intact but wipes out short-term memory. You can find your way around the house in which you've lived for fifty years, but move into an assisted-living facility and you're completely lost, as if in a maze. You can't remember which hallways you've already explored and which ones are new. What if you couldn't trace your steps back to the entrance of the building, because you couldn't remember any landmarks? You would panic, and perhaps freeze, maybe give up and sit in the same place all day until someone came to lead you back. This is exactly what happens to a person with Alzheimer's disease, an illness that interferes with memory, especially memory of place.

Alzheimer's usually occurs in people in their seventies and eighties, though it can appear earlier in some rare hereditary forms. It starts with mild impairment of short-term episodic memory—difficulty recalling recent events and new names— and gradually progresses, over nine or ten years, to a complete inability to know time and place or recognize friends and family. In later stages, Alzheimer patients may have difficulties with movement, such as walking, or may develop tremors. Eventually patients become stuporous and comatose, and because swallowing is also impaired, often die from choking or pneumonia.

An autopsy will reveal that the brain is severely shrunken, especially in areas involved in learning and memory—the temporal and parietal lobes and the frontal cortex. Within the temporal lobe, those areas essential to spatial memory are the most affected, among them the hippocampus and amygdala. The nerve cells in these areas have shriveled and died. Under the microscope, you can see patches of coagulated protein between the cells, and, inside the cells, tangles that look like hairballs. Pathologists call these *plaques and tangles,* and have found them to be a characteristic feature of Alzheimer's. The plaques are accumulations of a protein called *beta-amyloid;* the tangles are degenerated filaments that usually form a kind of skeleton inside the cell. These accumulate as a result of the action of several important enzymes, which break down the normal proteins in nerve cells and their surroundings and cause them to assume an abnormal shape. But plaques and tangles can also be seen in the brains of people who died from other causes, without any symptoms of memory loss or nerve damage. So other factors must be needed in Alzheimer's to bring on memory loss. Though the evidence is not conclusive, one of those factors is thought to be inflammation.

Under the microscope, brain tissue from Alzheimer's patients shows macrophage-like immune cells that live permanently in the brain. Called *glial cells,* they accumulate around the deposits of abnormal proteins, and spew out immune molecules as they gobble up the debris. The cells act as if they've encountered a foreign invader that needs to cleared. Except in this case it is the brain's own nerve cells—especially those clumps of degenerated beta-amyloid protein—that they are attacking with their own proteins, called *cytokines* or *interleukins.*

Inter plus *leukin,* in Latin, means "between white blood cells." When immunologists came up with the term, they thought the main job of these proteins was to help white blood cells communicate with each other. But it turned out that interleukins not only promote growth and division of immune cells, and help them make antibodies, and kill viruses—they also kill nerve cells. Though no one knows what makes proteins shrivel and nerve cells die in Alzheimer's disease, the inflammation that occurs around the plaques and tangles can certainly kill more nerve cells and could be a trigger that sets up a vicious cycle in the brain.

Why does Alzheimer's particularly affect the hippocampus and other parts of the brain important in memory of place? Some researchers believe that this may have something to do with wiring. In the course of the disease, the first part of the brain in which nerve cells die is the locus ceruleus, that brainstem region governing the stress response. The nerve cells in this region send long axon fibers directly to the hippocampus, where they release their adrenalin-like nerve chemical norepinephrine. This is how these two regions of the brain communicate. Although norepinephrine's main function is to allow the electrical impulse to jump from one nerve cell to another, it also has effects on immune cells. In the brain, it shuts off inflammation. When nerve cells in the locus ceruleus die, their axons die as well and cease to inject their anti-inflammatory norepinephrine into the hippocampus. According to this theory, if abnormal beta-amyloid accumulates, the immune cells in the area become overactive; when they don't shut off, inflammation escalates. And they kill additional nerve cells.

There is another conundrum in this illness that has long puzzled neurologists. In the early stages of Alzheimer's, there are clear impairments in memory before any pathological changes become evident. Why? It turns out that the same immune molecules which kill nerve cells also play a role in the formation of memories—especially those that involve place. It may be that these immune molecules impair nerve-cell function and memory formation even before the nerve cells die.

Try to remember what you were doing and the details of your surroundings the last time you had the flu, or an infection of any sort. It's hard to reconstruct the events and places that you experienced. Everything is a blur. Of the many sorts of memories you might form—memory of passing time, of events, of place— illness affects them all, but it especially affects memory of place. Several scientists working on different continents contributed a great deal to our understanding of how these immune molecules affect memory.

At the base of the Front Range, in the Colorado Rockies, the Flatirons form a landmark that is impossible to forget. They're large, flat cliffs that stick straight up out of the ground. Dating from the geological period when these mountains thrust upward and turned the underlying bedrock on its end, they are named for the shape they resemble: the flat bottom of a household iron. They are located just west of Boulder, where Steve Maier and his wife, Linda Watkins, teach and do neuroscience research at the University of Colorado. Compact and wiry, the couple are avid sports enthusiasts who bike, run, ski, and scuba dive, pursuing all of the activities with the style and dedication of Olympic athletes.

In 1994 and 1995 Maier and Watkins, along with two other researchers, one in France and another in Canada, proved that one important route through which immune molecules signal the brain is the vagus nerve—the thick cable of nerve fibers that extends through the spinal cord to the brain. It is this nerve that can make you faint when you are punched in the solar plexus. It is the same nerve that lowers blood pressure and slows the heart during meditation and relaxation. And it is the reason you feel the way you do when you are sick.

The ways we feel and act when we are ailing are called, not surprisingly, *sickness behaviors*. We're all familiar with these: loss of appetite, diminished interest in the outside world, decreased interest in sex, a reluctance to move, a desire to rest, sleepiness, depressed mood, impaired ability to think clearly, and loss of memory. These symptoms are not caused by fever. Rather, the immune molecules the body produces to fight infection cause both the fever and all of the other changes.

When I asked Steve Maier why he did this research, he emphatically answered, "If you put the question to your grandmother correctly, she would tell you that there has to be a way for immune molecules to get to the brain to make you *feel* sick. These molecules were in the literature, but none of the blood-borne mechanisms made sense as the only way for them to get to the brain. We and Robert Dantzer showed that the vagus nerve was the way the signal got there, but really it was Dwight Nance who figured that one out."

Nance, a neuroanatomist whose specialty is the vagus nerve, was a professor at the University of Winnipeg in 1993, when he presented his then still-unpublished work at a psychoneuro-immunology meeting in Boulder. He showed that a tiny area deep in the brain stem called the *nucleus of the tractus solitarius* (NTS) was the switching station in the brain for signals from the abdomen.

As Nance later recounted the events to me: "Linda and Steve were at that meeting. They cornered me at the bar and basically began to pick my brain." Watkins and Maier described the work they were doing on sickness behaviors, and their puzzlement over how the sickness signals got to the brain when they injected bits of bacteria into the abdomen of a rat. "With my background in feeding behavior," Nance continued, "I knew it had to be the liver. The liver is richly innervated by the vagus nerve. All their data led to the liver. Basically, they came to me and I said, 'Dig here!'"

Watkins and Maier followed Nance's advice. They cut the vagus above the liver, and injected either interleukin-1 or endo-toxin into the rats' bellies. The animals acted perfectly normally; they did not act ill and did not develop fever, unlike rats whose vagus nerve was left intact. This proved that besides regulating the rhythms of the heart and the stress response, as Julian Thayer and Ary Goldberger had shown when they studied people's responses to music, the vagus nerve was also the main link for communicating sickness signals from the abdomen to the brain.

The problem still remained: How could the immune molecules possibly turn on electrical activity in the vagus nerve? For immunologists and neurobiologists at the time, this seemed like heresy. They thought that only nerve chemicals could turn on nerves. It was Maier and Watkins' co-worker Lisa Goehler who came up with the key experiment to figure this out. Goehler was a neuroanatomist at the University of Colorado, Boulder, and an expert in the *autonomic nervous system*—the part of the nervous system that includes nerves like the vagus, which supply the gut and heart and skin, to make you sweat, slow your heartbeat, and give you stomach cramps when you are stressed or after a meal. She was one of a small group of scientists at Boulder, including Maier and Watkins and Moni Fleshner (who was doing her studies on exercise and the immune system), who would meet weekly to brainstorm. They talked about results that puzzled them and discussed the scientific papers they had read that might provide some answers.

They wanted to identify which cells in the vagus nerve were binding the immune molecules. Goehler predicted it would be nerve cells. Borrowing a well-known method in neuroanatomy, in which a nerve chemical's antagonist was routinely used to measure such binding, rather than the nerve chemical itself, Goehler used the antagonist of the immune molecule interleukin-1 (IL-1) to see where it attached. She injected the dye-labeled molecule into the abdomen of rats and examined the vagus nerve. When she looked under the microscope, she had her answer.

The molecule did indeed bind to the vagus nerve, but not, it seemed, to the nerve fibers themselves. The cells that lit up under the microscope were buried in clusters inside bulges along the nerve. Some of the nerve fibers even touched these mystery cells, just as they might connect to another nerve fiber. The cells had a name, but until then no one knew what these cells did. They were called *paraganglia cells.*

Puzzled by this finding, Goehler consulted with a German colleague, the neuroanatomist Hans Rudy Berthoud, who was doing research on paraganglia. He told her they were not nerve cells but *chemosensory cells*—cells whose main job is to sense chemicals in the environment. So Goehler had found that one of the chemicals in the environment that these cells sense is the immune molecule interleukin-1. Their job is to tell the brain that there is infection or inflammation in the abdomen. When you are sick with appendicitis, for example, immune molecules released from the site of infection send signals to the brain by binding to those cells that sit alongside the vagus nerve. This stimulates electrical firing of the nerve that relays to the NTS, the brain center that Dwight Nance had discovered.

Around the time that Watkins and Maier made their discovery, Robert Dantzer, a scientist from Bordeaux, showed that the vagus nerve goes one step further in signaling sickness to the brain. Dantzer is an erudite and charming Frenchman whose deep velvety voice evokes the great French chansonniers of the twentieth century. A veterinarian by training, he has thought long and hard about the nature of sickness behaviors. He was among the first to use this phrase to denote the constellation of symptoms that all animals exhibit when they are ill.

Dantzer claims it was the work of the Swiss researcher Hugo Besedovsky, showing that the brain's stress response was activated when interleukin-1 was injected into the abdomen, which got him started. Mainly because he didn't believe it. He injected IL-1, at doses used by Besedovsky, into animals and tested several behaviors that are impaired during illness—behaviors with which he was very familiar from his stress research. One was taste aversion, a sensitive indicator of stress and appetite. Another was social exploration, which, like appetite, decreases during illness. He found that the immune molecule impaired them all. He was finally convinced that Besedovsky was right. Integrating his results with the findings of other researchers, he proposed that during illness the brain orchestrates a set of motivational behaviors which protect the animal by helping it conserve its energy to fight infection. When we exhibit these sickness behaviors, we are not just passively withdrawing from the world—we are actively seeking withdrawal so as to preserve our physiological resources.

The logical next step was to ask what was causing the behaviors: Was it IL-1 in the abdomen or IL-1 in the brain? The problem was familiar to Dantzer from his previous research with other molecules made both in the brain and in the rest of the body: How does the message get from the periphery to the brain? Dantzer did a simple experiment, injecting IL-1 either into the abdomen or into the brain, and then measuring IL-1 in the other organ. The technologies for measuring small amounts of these molecules were then still very crude. It took him a year to set up the technique, but he finally proved that when IL-1 is injected into the abdomen of rats, interleukin-1 is also produced in the brain and sickness behaviors ensue.

Like Maier and Watkins, Dantzer was impressed with Dwight Nance's study on the vagus nerve. "Nance had shown that the NTS processes and organizes information from the gut in a very complex way. It's more than a simple relay station," he told me when we talked one afternoon at a recent meeting. Dantzer asked an associate, then technician Rose-Marie Bluthé, to perform the same experiments they had been doing on sickness behaviors, but this time to cut the vagus nerve before injecting IL-1 into the abdomen of the rats. Bluthé, a skilled animal surgeon, knew a great deal about agronomy. She also had a role model in her mother, who had become a technician in the biological sciences after meeting and marrying a German Jewish refugee (Rose-Marie's father) while working in the French Resistance during World War II. A devout Roman Catholic, Bluthé told me that when she was a child, she and her mother had made many pilgrimages to Lourdes, the healing sanctuary in southwest France.

She recalled how excited Dantzer was in planning these experiments, and how proud he was of her skill at performing the delicate surgery on which their success depended. The results were positive. Dantzer and Bluthé found that not only did sickness behaviors fail to appear in the animals whose nerve had been cut, but IL-1 was no longer made in the animals' brains. The baton in the relay race of immune signals coursing to the brain during illness turned out to be the immune molecule itself. They had found that it is made first in the gut, during infection or inflammation, and then in the brain, once the electrical signals have traveled there via the vagus nerve.

These discoveries raised a whole series of new questions about what else such immune molecules were doing in the brain. Is it brain interleukin-1 that causes sickness behaviors and makes us less able to remember places when we're ill? Could it be that immune molecules in the brain interfere with learning and the formation of memories, especially memories of place?

Evidence was accumulating that memory and thought processes were impaired in Alzheimer's disease and AIDS dementia. The same was true in inflammatory conditions like autoimmune diseases and in infections, where immune molecules were elevated in the blood. It had also been reported that when patients were undergoing cancer chemotherapy and immune molecules were administered to boost their immune systems, their memory became impaired. New research had shown, too, that immune molecules in the brain could kill nerve cells.

To Watkins and Maier, the evidence was overwhelming: immune molecules like interleukin-1 could well be having an effect on memory. But Maier predicted that these molecules did not affect all types of memory equally: their main effect would be on forming memories of place. Perhaps being sick interfered with making the connection between a particular place and the thing that is learned in that place— i.e., contextual memory. In fact, old rat experiments in the taste-aversion field had shown that illness interferes with memory of elements of place—a light or a sound—but not of a taste. Maier reasoned that it's of no adaptive use to associate sickness with the place you got sick, but it *is* highly useful to associate taste with sickness, because it was probably something you ate that made you sick. When you're sick, the brain has to take the hippocampus offline, so you don't associate place with sickness. This had to be why, Maier reasoned, those immune molecules bound most densely in the hippocampus, the part of the brain important in memory of place.

Ruth Barrientos, a young postdoctoral student in Maier and Watkins' lab, was assigned the project of testing this hypothesis. A tall woman with satiny black hair and olive-colored skin, she had come a long way from her birthplace in Bolivia. Always fascinated by studies of learning and memory, she had convinced me, when I was her supervisor at NIH, to let her set up a water maze to test memory differences in arthritis-prone rats. She was a tough negotiator, and didn't take no for an answer, even when I insisted that I knew nothing about such behavioral tests. She found experts in behavioral research who could help her, investigated how much the apparatus would cost, and located space in the animal facility where the apparatus could be placed.

At Boulder, Barrientos trained rats to associate a particular context with a mild electrical shock. The environments she used were simple: one was the inside of a black ice bucket with a lid that she used for carrying the rats, and the other was the inside of an empty white ice chest which she had fitted with a light bulb so the rats could see. After becoming familiar with each environment, the rats were given a very mild, brief shock through the floor of the white ice chest. This procedure is called *fear-conditioning* and is used in many types of studies to define the brain's fear circuits and to develop treatments for anxiety disorders. Anyone who has taken a pet dog or cat to the vet in a carrier cage has effectively done this experiment. After one or two trips, the dog or cat will associate the carrier with the experience of going to the vet. Once it learns this, you'll have a difficult time coaxing it into the carrier the next time. Covering it with a blanket may be the only solution. This works because without the benefit of vision, the animal can't see the inside of the carrier that it has learned to associate with the negative experience.

After training the animals, Barrientos injected either inter-leukin-1 or a tiny volume of plain salt water (saline solution) directly into the hippocampus of the rats after they had learned the context but before they received the shock. The rats who received only saline showed behaviors typical of fear: freezing in place, refusing to explore. Those who received the interleukin-1 showed fewer of these behaviors, and acted more like the control rats who had never received a shock. The interleukin had kept the fearful memory from being cemented to memory of the place.

The process also works the other way around. Nobel laureate Eric Kandel, a psychiatrist and neuroscientist at Columbia University, showed that rats and mice can learn to associate a particular context with safety, if they repeatedly find that the negative experience does not occur in a particular place. Context can evoke other kinds of positive memories too, including memories of desire. Drug addicts will often relapse when they find themselves in the surroundings where they became addicted: they learned to associate the context with the rush they experienced from the drugs, and being in that place will revive their cravings. This happens in smokers, too—they feel the urge to light up a cigarette when entering a place where they had routinely smoked before.

Animals can learn to associate a place with an addictive drug like morphine. The test method, first performed in 1940 with chimpanzees, is called *conditioned place preference*. Eventually the experimental design was modified and applied to mice and rats. In such studies, rats are given injections of the addicting drug in one chamber, and an injection of saline in another. Drugs that have been studied in this way include cocaine, morphine, methamphetamine, nicotine, alcohol, caffeine, and cannabis. All of these activate the brain's dopamine reward pathways and produce the pleasurable feeling that addicts crave.

The different contexts that the rats learn to associate with the reward can be very complex: the colors and patterns on the walls, the textures of the floor, the lighting, the sounds, and the smells. The wallpaper of the test chambers may be horizontally or vertically striped; the floors either cork or tile; and the lighting of various colors and brightnesses. The rat learns to associate the addictive drug only with the chamber in which it received the drug, and only with the specific features of the place. When it is presented with a choice between two differently decorated chambers, the addicted animal will choose to enter the one that it has connected with the drug, and not the other, even if there is no drug around. Animals who are not addicted show no preference for either place.

An animal can learn to associate a place with any reward—drugs, food, water, exercise on a running wheel, or sex with a receptive mate. A rat trained in this way will crave the particular reward in the particular place, and it will spend more time in the chamber it associates with the reward than it does in any other space. The greater the pleasure it derives from a given reward, the longer it will spend in the chamber. The extent to which it searches also depends on its motivational state. A hungry rat will spend more time in the context it associates with food; a thirsty rat will spend more time in the context it associates with water; and a rat deprived of sex will spend more time in the chamber where it mated. But if the animal is sated, it will show no place preference.

Watkins and Maier also tested the effects of immune molecules on this type of association. They found they could block animals' ability to form positive associations of reward and place with drugs that prevent activation of glial cells, the immune cells in the brain that produce immune molecules such as interleukins. Such drugs also reduced the rats' symptoms of withdrawal from addictive drugs. This showed that immune molecules, released from activated glial cells in the hippocampus, play an important part in drug addiction and withdrawal, especially when linked to memory of place. This discovery could aid in the development of drugs to treat relapses into addiction.

All these experiments proved that immune molecules such as interleukin-1 affect learning and memory of place when an animal is sick. But the question remained whether immune molecules can affect learning and memory in *healthy* organisms. Half a world away from Colorado, in Marburg, Germany, Hugo Besedovsky and his wife, Adriana del Rey, were exploring this question.

The town of Marburg could have come straight out of Disneyland—all that's missing is Cinderella and the prince. Indeed, this is where the Brothers Grimm collected their fairy tales. Medieval half-timbered houses, some decorated with Gothic script, line the cobbled streets that climb to the hilltop castle above the town. The princes who lived in this castle were the rulers of the surrounding lands, and the townspeople were their indentured servants who worked the farms.

In the nineteenth and twentieth centuries, the University of Marburg, founded in 1527, developed a reputation for excellence in the field of infectious diseases. The Marburg virus, a disease endemic to Africa that causes rapid death from massive bleeding, was discovered here. It received its name in 1967, after a terrible outbreak occurred in the town when laboratory workers were exposed to an infected monkey. The University of Marburg recruited Hugo Besedovsky and Adriana del Rey after they proved that immune molecules such as interleukin-1, which are released by immune cells during infection, signal the brain and activate its stress response.

Adriana del Rey, born in Argentina, came from a long line of strong and independent women. Her grandmother had been one of the first women to obtain a doctorate in philosophy from the University of Salamanca in Spain, at the end of the nineteenth century, and had emigrated to South America after her marriage. Besedovsky was likewise Argentinean; his grandparents had emigrated from the Ukraine to escape the anti-Semitic persecutions of the late nineteenth century. His father was a physician who often took young Hugo with him on his rounds.

Besedovsky and del Rey left Argentina for Switzerland, settling first in Davos, a center of the heliotherapy movement which had inspired twentieth-century modernist architects, and also the setting of Thomas Mann's novel *The Magic Mountain,* about life in a TB sanatorium. They then spent fifteen years in Basel, an immunology research capital, proving their theory that immune molecules could trigger the brain's stress response. The idea was inconceivable to immunologists and neurobiologists. How and why could the immune system trigger the brain's stress response? Researchers thought that immune molecules, too large to cross from blood into the brain, couldn't possibly have this effect.

The new concept was not so far from Hans Selye's theories of a generalized sickness response that called into play the brain's stress center. Except Selye didn't have the benefit of knowing that when he injected material into rats and they became ill, they were most likely producing interleukins. Besedovsky and del Rey eventually published their findings in *Science* magazine in

1987. The study, performed in collaboration with a team of researchers from the Netherlands, proved beyond a shadow of a doubt that an immune molecule, interleukin-1, activates the hypothalamus, the part of the brain that controls the stress response.

Besedovsky and del Rey went on to ask what other effects immune molecules might have on brain function. They especially wanted to know whether interleukin-1 could influence memory. By the time they started their experiments, technologies had become available to study not only whole-brain memory function in rats, but also what happens to single nerve cells when a memory is being made.

They knew of Dantzer's work showing that interleukin-1 was expressed in the brain during sickness behaviors. They also knew the studies of Maier and Watkins, who had shown that when the vagus nerve was cut, sickness behaviors were prevented. Many years before, del Rey and Besedovsky had found that electrical activity in the brain increased after dead bacteria were injected into a rat's abdomen. And it was known that high concentrations of receptors for interleukin-1 were present in memory centers in the brain, especially the hippocampus. Putting these pieces of information together, they reasoned that the immune molecules expressed in the brain after the exposure to bacteria could be causing the increase in electrical activity. This theory would be difficult to prove in the whole animal, so they chose to test whether interleukin-1 could trigger electrical activity in nerve cells in brain-tissue slices maintained in culture dishes. The test system they used, called *long-term potentiation*, measures a type of electrical activity important in creating nerve connections during learning and memory.

Several things happen to your brain cells when you learn or remember something. If a first experience is just a brief encounter, a nerve cell starts firing electrical impulses. But each time you repeat a task and learn it, nerve cells sprout new connections, like tiny fingers, that grow out to touch one another across synaptic space. It used to be thought that after infancy, nerve cells stopped growing. But Eric Kandel, studying the lowly sea slug, proved that nerve cells continue to grow and make new connections during the process of learning. In October 2000 he received the Nobel Prize for this discovery. Kandel likes to begin his lectures by saying that at the end of the talk—if you've been listening hard—you will leave with a few more nerve-cell connections than you had when you came in. We now know that these connections are constantly forming and re-forming, sometimes in the course of minutes. What makes these connections more permanent is still a mystery.

Before you can see any anatomical changes in a nerve cell, you can measure the changes in its electrical activity that occur with learning. Each time a nerve cell encounters the same stimulus—as happens with repeated exposure to any event—it fires off many trains of electrical impulses. In the laboratory, researchers can mimic this effect by applying trains of repeated electrical impulses to various brain regions. The repetition strengthens the connections between nerve cells. You can do the same to slices of the hippocampus that have been removed from a rat or mouse and placed in a tissue-culture dish. The slices will continue to function electrically and biochemically for several hours. Applying bursts of electrical impulses to the slices, researchers can measure the resulting biochemical changes, and gain a sense of what happens during learning as the connections become more long-lasting. This process is what scientists call *long-term potentiation*.

Besedovsky and del Rey found that when nerve cells in the hippocampal slices were exposed to such electrical impulses, interleukin-1 genes turn on and started making interleukin-1. When a drug that blocked interleukin-1 was added to the slices, electrical impulses disappeared. It was like a two-way switch: electrical impulses turned on interleukin-1, and interleukin-1 seemed to be needed to keep the impulses flowing. When the researchers measured electrical firing in the hippocampus of awake, moving rats in which they had implanted a brain electrode, the drug that blocked interleukin-1 also blocked electrical firing in the hippocampus. It seemed that interleukin-1 was needed to maintain the basic cellular processes that nerve cells undergo when a memory is being formed.

Watkins and Maier and others had shown that high concentrations of interleukin-1 can impair memory of place when we are sick. Besedovsky and del Rey showed that this same molecule is necessary for maintenance of learning and memory under normal circumstances. This difference is often seen in biological systems. A molecule when present in excess (as occurs in illness) can do harm; yet when present in smaller amounts, it is essential for normal functions. Experiments like those of Watkins and Maier and Besedovsky and del Rey tell us that interleukin-1 plays an important role in memory formation both during illness and in health.

This may be the reason that in Alzheimer's patients, where there is inflammation in the brain and immune molecules are produced in excess, deficits in memory occur even before nerve cells die. The immune molecules released by activated brain immune cells interfere with the nerve cells' processes of memory formation. It is likely that this is also happening in your brain when you are sick with an inflammatory or infectious disease and are producing immune molecules to fight infection. If you are then sent from one department to another in the hospital, your ability to form a memory of the route will be impaired. You may be less able to recognize the landmarks along the way. And if you don't recognize where you are, you might lose your way and become anxious.

Why not, then, design hospitals and healthcare facilities taking these scientific principles into account? They could be designed in such a way as to facilitate navigation and reduce anxiety. As Walt Disney and Frank Gehry demonstrated, it is possible to design places that trigger anxiety and fear, or design them to make people feel happy and secure. By taking people from fear to comfort, the works of Disney and Gehry promote feelings of well-being. Most hospitals today instill fear, but they don't inspire hope. More than anything, a person who is ill needs an environment that fosters calm and comfort as a means to healing. The spaces around us can and should do this.

The architect Charles Jencks, when interviewed in a PBS television documentary directed by Sydney Pollack, said that Gehry "is committed to a notion of an architecture that relates to healing." Jencks should know. Gehry designed a tranquil, restorative refuge in memory of Jencks's wife, Maggie Keswick, who died of cancer. This small, whimsical, modernist building, reminiscent of a thatched-roof cottage, is set in the rolling countryside near Dundee, Scotland, and is one of a series of Maggie's Centres designed by master architects. It is filled with places for reflection, and provides views of the peaceful hills all around.

Architects who specialize in healthcare design have begun taking these principles into account in the planning of hospitals and healthcare facilities. One such place, known as "The Village," is located at the Waveny Care Center in New Canaan, Connecticut. Architects from the firm Reese, Lower, Patrick & Scott designed this center specifically for individuals with dementia. It incorporates features that serve as prostheses to aid failing memories, just as canes and walkers act as prostheses to aid failing legs. In the residents' rooms, the architects angled the beds so that there are direct sightlines to the toilet in the bathroom and to the window, which opens onto a view of the outdoors. So the residents have no need to remember where the bathroom is—it's in plain view. They can find their way to the bathroom on their own, and thus remain independent longer than they would in standard facilities.

Residents spend most of their day not in their rooms, but on the center's gently curving, glass-roofed Main Street. This indoor space, flooded with natural light, looks and feels as though it is outdoors. It is lined with what appear to be two-story red-brick or wooden buildings; there are colorful awnings, flower boxes, faux wrought-iron balconies. These serve as visual cues and landmarks that tell residents where they are. Other landmarks are visible along the street. The clock above one of the elevators is large and round; its black hands and numbers stand out against a white background. An outdoor enclosed garden at one end of the street is distinctly different from the indoor view at the opposite end.

These landmarks orient the residents, who can wander safely on their own. The street is lined with storefronts, bakeries, ice cream parlors, cafés, and park benches, and is monitored by attendants. During the day, residents can sit and watch street performers, or participate in organized events. In the evening, old-style street lamps light the space. The outdoors is clearly visible from most places in the Waveny Center, including the rooms and eating areas, to help the occupants orient themselves with respect not only to place but also to time of day and season.

This unique feature, Main Street, came about as a result of the client's request to the architects when the center was being designed. He had observed that most of the residents came from New Canaan and similar Victorian-era towns in Connecticut, where they had enjoyed spending time in the town centers. He felt that creating a space that resembled the Main Streets they were used to might make the residents feel more at home. When the architects heard this, Disneyland's Main Street immediately came to mind. And so they incorporated many of the features of Disney's Main Street into the design. Disney would certainly be glad to know that his concepts have inspired some of the most successful and advanced assisted-living residences in the country. They are improving quality of life for the elderly, and helping them to cope with memory loss and isolation.

Some of the beneficial effects of this environment may stem from the rich and varied experiences that the residents encounter throughout the day. They may also come from exercise, as Moni Fleshner demonstrated in her studies of rats and mice. Other researchers have proved that enriched environments incorporating running wheels and toys can reverse learning impairments in mice genetically engineered to develop memory impairments, nerve-cell death, and brain atrophy—conditions that resemble the brain changes that occur in diseases like Alzheimer's. Such mice not only were able to access old memories, but also sprouted new nerve connections in the hippocampus; the mice housed in barren, empty cages did not. It's still unclear how much of the benefit of these environments comes from exercise and how much from the mental stimulation provided by the toys and activities in them, but there is no question that enriched environments coupled with moderate exercise can help to preserve memory and improve mood.

Indeed, there are places in the world where the experience of entering a place seems to have an almost miraculous ability to soothe anxiety and despair, and to cure physical ills as well. New research is beginning to reveal the mechanisms of such cures.

8

HEALING THOUGHT AND
HEALING PRAYER

If there is one place on earth where you can step from inside out—from indoors to outdoors, and from inside yourself to the world you share with others—it is Lourdes, in the foothills of the French Pyrenees. In 1858, a fourteen-year-old peasant girl named Bernadette Soubirous saw visions of the Virgin Mary at a spring in Lourdes, and ever since then the town has been a center of healing. Each year it attracts approximately six million visitors and eighty thousand ailing pilgrims. What is it about this place that draws them there?

The story of Bernadette, her visions, and their healing power has inspired people throughout the world. According to the legend, the girl was washing clothes beside the Gave de Pau, a river near her village, when the Virgin Mary appeared to her above a spring that welled up from the rocks in a grotto at the water's edge. The Virgin commanded Bernadette to drink the water from the spring—a dirty, muddy source where townsfolk threw their trash. Bernadette prayed and obeyed.

At first, no one believed Bernadette when she described the experience. But her visions persisted—eighteen in all. Finally, a woman from a neighboring village who had been suffering from a dislocated shoulder came to visit Bernadette at the spring. Again, the Virgin appeared. The woman plunged her arm into the icy waters and was miraculously healed. News of the cure spread throughout France. Bernadette convinced the bishop that the visions were real and obtained his promise that a church would be built on the site. To this day, people have continued to visit the shrine, to drink the water, bathe in the spring, pray, and be healed.

The collection of mostly Belle Epoque buildings hugs the slopes of three hills that form a bowl-shaped valley. Driving south toward the Pyrenees from nearby Pau and Tarbes, you cross a richly cultivated plain that suddenly gives way to the mountains. Entering the town by car is no small feat, for pilgrims crowd the narrow, winding streets. Their pace is slow. Many are on crutches or in wheelchairs or being supported by friends and family. Often they pause at the hundreds of shops and stalls selling religious paraphernalia. In the tangle of streets, there is only one route to your goal. As if on a treasure hunt, you follow the signs and arrows pointing to the grotto where Bernadette saw her visions.

At the base of the hill is the Gave de Pau, a broad, swift-flowing stream colored a milky turquoise from the glacial melt that supplies it. Next to the river is a parking lot. From this unlikely spot, a paved monument to modern transportation, you glimpse the cathedral rising against its mountain backdrop. The valley traps the early morning mist, which in turn traps the sunlight and gives the air a shimmering quality that bathes the river, the church, and all who enter there.

As you walk from the parking lot to the small footbridge that leads across the river to the cathedral square, you see an amazing sight. Hundreds of uniformed nurses are pushing patients in wheelchairs or on stretchers toward the cathedral. They wear blue-and-white pinstriped dresses with white pinafores, or plain white uniforms, or striking blue-and-red capes emblazoned with the Maltese Cross of the Order of Saint John. It is not only nurses who help the sick. Nearly every patient has at least one helper. Some pilgrims who are unable to walk are seated in bright-blue buggies drawn by *brancardiers,* men in blue uniforms specifically trained to transport the sick. Others walk in groups, their leaders holding banners proclaiming their towns of origin—places in France, Ireland, England, Italy, Germany, the Philippines, Australia, the United States, and more.

They are all heading toward the plaza surrounding the cathedral to pray, to place flowers at the base of the Vièrge Couronnée (a statue of the crowned Virgin Mary facing the Cathedral), and to drink the water from the spring—the one from which Bernadette drank at the behest of the Virgin. Now the water is piped from the grotto and available from dozens of taps, where people line up to fill their vessels. If you didn't bring a container, you can purchase one—anything from a tiny glass bottle decorated with images of Bernadette and the Virgin, to a fifty-gallon plastic container you could ship home.

Just beyond the taps lies the grotto itself. The pilgrims line up to file past it and the spring, which is now covered with protective glass and which bubbles up to the floor of this unassuming limestone cavity, only nine meters deep and three meters high. Above it is a smaller opening where the Virgin Mary appeared. This now contains a statue of the Virgin, and a wild rose bush that is said to have sprouted from the rock when she first appeared. Long tapers burn on a stand beneath the statue, pointing the way to an alley of candles where the faithful can light their own. These range from slender tapers that cost one euro, to enormous candles the size of logs, needing two strong men to carry them. Here the wax of decades and the condensing mist make the path slippery, but the heat from the hundreds of burning candles warms the passers-by.

Beyond the candles are the baths. Pilgrims wait in a covered area, before they are ushered inside in groups and immersed in tubs of water from the spring. While they wait, they sing songs, sometimes accompanied by guitars. All are joined in a common purpose: to pray and to be healed.

As you make your way across the plaza from one station to the next, you step into a different kind of healing space—the one that exists between two devout individuals. The clergyman Maurice Gardès, who spends a great deal of time in this intimate space, was once a physicist. He began his career studying particles that he could measure but could not see, then turned to the study of beliefs that he could not measure. Today he is the archbishop of Auch, the diocese neighboring Lourdes. Dressed in a black clerical suit and white collar, with a large silver Cross suspended from his neck, he is instantly recognizable as a leader of the church.

In 2006, I accompanied him to Lourdes. He could not go five paces without being greeted by pilgrims, mothers holding babies, invalids in wheelchairs, groups of matrons giggling shyly like schoolgirls. They spoke Chinese, Italian, Spanish, Portuguese, French, English, and a dozen other languages. All solemnly requested that he bless them and their loved ones, as well as the vials of water they would be bringing home. He listened patiently to the stories, and with a warm and loving look blessed each pilgrim. In that moment, in the space between him and the believer, a tiny oasis of peace and calm was created amid the throng.

On a Sunday, you can attend Mass at the grotto, in the open air, or you can go to one of the many churches on the site: the old cathedral, the crown-shaped sanctuary beneath it, the tiny crypt beneath them, or the vast underground cathedral across the way. When empty, this modern church looks like a dimly lit, low-ceilinged sports arena, whose concrete walls are adorned with backlit stained-glass murals depicting the Stations of the Cross. When full, it is completely transformed, holding several thousand people. Many nurses attend the service, either with their patients or in groups, wearing the distinctive uniforms of their healing orders. Dozens of bishops and archbishops come from around the world to participate in the Mass. They give Communion in the aisles and in the concourse around the periphery of the space, before joining the procession out of the church at the end of the service.

Reaching out to strangers is accepted and even welcomed here. A father pushes a young girl, about ten years old, in her wheelchair. She is unable to move her legs and has limited use of her hands. She seems overwhelmed by the crowds; the look in her eyes is vacant. Two pilgrims in hiking gear notice the girl. They approach her at the point in the Mass when the bishop invites the congregation to shake hands with their neighbors and say "Peace be with you." One of the pilgrims reaches out to the child, who looks at him confused. Without hesitation or embarrassment, he takes her hand in his and shows her how to squeeze it. She grasps it, all the while looking into his face. He nods and smiles. She continues clasping his hand and her face lights up, suffused with joy. As her father pushes her wheelchair through the crowd, her beatific smile persists. She seems to have been transported to some place of wonder in her mind. And even if only for a little while, this interchange has clearly relieved her pain.

The Mass is only one of many opportunities for visitors to pray and show their love of the Virgin Mary. Most events take place outdoors, in the square between the cathedral and the Crowned Virgin. Every afternoon, the pilgrims assemble for a procession that will lead them over the bridge and into the square in front of the cathedral. They arrange themselves in groups, one member of each group holding a colorful banner identifying their town and country of origin. People mill around, chatting or resting on the benches beside the stream until the bells of the cathedral signal the appointed hour. Then the people stand and quietly move into their groups, helped by Lourdes' staff and the brancardiers, who make sure the sickest are up front. The process is surprisingly quiet and orderly, considering that it involves thousands of people. They fall into formation within a few minutes. It's like some graceful military drill.

When the bells ring out at five o'clock, the procession moves slowly forward. The bishop leads, holding aloft a beautifully ornate silver vessel containing the Host, which represents the body of Christ. Amid a flood of music, bells and chimes, the bishop chants a Latin prayer which is broadcast throughout the area. The choir echoes him as he walks toward the footbridge, surrounded by his entourage of bishops, many visiting from far-off lands. The procession follows him across the bridge and into the square. First come the standard-bearers, waving their flags high. Then come the sick on stretchers, in wheelchairs, and in the little blue carts. Troops of nurses follow in their signature uniforms. Finally come those on foot, each delegation holding high its banner.

The parade has a joyous, festive air. The banners make you think of a medieval tournament. You almost expect to see a battalion of knights in shining armor bringing up the rear on horseback. The procession moves in fits and starts, to accommodate the ailing and the disabled. At each stop, nurses lean over their charges, adjusting the patients' sweaters, propping their pillows, holding water to their lips, and looking into their faces with warmth and love. Gradually, every inch of space between the Crowned Virgin and the cathedral fills up with people. The bishop blesses the faithful and says a short prayer.

Remarkable as this sight is, it is not the most striking ceremony that takes place at Lourdes. Every evening, as the sun is setting, the pilgrims assemble for a candlelight procession. Each holds a long taper, purchased for a couple of euros, and in the deepening darkness all that is visible is the flickering light of thousands of candles. The space seems almost as bright as day. As the procession passes, you can glimpse the faces in the flames' soft light, suffused with peace and joy. The pilgrims are happy to be part of this assemblage, to be in this place, members of a community with a shared purpose, achieving their dreams.

Watching from the grand stone staircase that curves around the cathedral, you may be struck by the resemblance between Lourdes and Disney's Magic Kingdom—where people likewise flock from all over the world, where crowds are shepherded in snaking, switch-back lines, where people buy mementos in little shops, where a large plaza is laid out beneath a hilltop castle. But this Kingdom is not for amusement. This one has very real and powerful effects on bodies in need of healing.

There have been sixty-seven officially acknowledged miracle cures at Lourdes since Bernadette Soubirous first saw her visions of the Virgin Mary. And every week there are more visitors who claim that they, too, have been miraculously healed. When I visited, the physician who determines whether there is a medical explanation for a cure was Dr. Patrick Theillier, head of the Lourdes Medical Bureau. He is charged with studying each possible miracle in depth—interviewing the patients, examining their pathology reports, and following up for at least five years to watch for recurrences. Once Dr. Theillier and the Medical Bureau have certified the cure, it must be reviewed by the highest secular authority, the International Medical Committee. If these bodies conclude that medical science cannot explain the cure, the case is passed on to the Catholic church, which makes the final judgment as to whether a miracle has occurred.

When asked about these cases, Dr. Theillier touches his trim gray beard and leans back in his chair. His thoughtful blue eyes seem to visualize the patients as he describes them. Prior to the 1950s, the majority of cures deemed miraculous involved people with tuberculosis. But individuals with cancer, bone infections, arthritis, and other diseases were judged to be healed as well. After tuberculosis drugs were developed in the latter part of the twentieth century, the types of illnesses deemed miraculously cured changed. Nowadays, most are in the category of autoimmune and inflammatory diseases, such as multiple sclerosis, inflammatory bowel disease, and rheumatoid arthritis, though tumors and heart disease are also on the list.

Typically, patients who experience these cures feel something the moment they join in one of the rituals at Lourdes. Often such moments occur in the baths, when the patients are touched by the water of the spring. The testimonials are remarkably consistent: patients recount that at that instant, well before there is any visible evidence of a cure, they are overcome with a profound and powerful emotion, a sense of joy and inner peace.

One recent cure was that of Jean-Pierre Bély, who suffered from multiple sclerosis, a disease in which the immune system attacks the brain. In 1984, at the age of forty-eight, Bély began to experience numbness and tingling in his legs, painful cramps at night, and difficulty walking. X-rays showed brain lesions typical of multiple sclerosis. He developed numbness in his right arm, violent headaches, and mild incontinence. Despite a variety of therapies, including conventional treatment with high-dose steroids and nonconventional treatment with African herbal medicines, he continued to deteriorate. He developed paralysis in his legs, rigidity and spasms in his muscles, dizziness, severe incontinence, and ringing in his ears.

In multiple sclerosis, immune cells attack nerve fibers in the brain and spinal cord and destroy them with antibodies and immune molecules that usually target invading viruses or bacteria, organisms foreign to the body. The inflammation in the brain can come in waves. The patient may feel perfectly well after an attack, and be struck down again months or years later. The disease can also be unremitting, progressing steadily to paralysis, as in Bély's case. Medical treatments rely on suppressing the immune system so that it ceases to attack the body. But once the damage has been done and scar tissue replaces healthy tissue, there is little chance that the patient will regain function.

On October 9, 1987, Bély came to Lourdes, deathly ill. After receiving Extreme Unction and the Last Rites, he felt (as he says in his testimony) a powerful sensation of "liberation and inner peace." He was overcome by a feeling of cold that became increasingly intense, almost painful, so that he needed extra blankets and hot water bottles. Then he fell into a stupor. This was followed by an intense warmth that spread throughout his body, starting in his toes and moving up through his feet, legs, hips, and spine.

He was seized by the urge to get up. He sat up, on the edge of his bed, surprised at his ability. He began to feel sensation in his fingers and skin. During Mass that day, he found he was able to shake a handkerchief without pain and with suppleness in his previously rigid muscles, which surprised him even more. The next night, after a period of deep sleep, Bély awoke suddenly at 3:00 A.M. when he heard the basilica's chimes. A voice in his head told him, "Go on, get up and walk!" Astonished, he got up and walked—for the first time in three years.

Though Bély's case was declared an unexplained cure by the Lourdes Medical Bureau and a miracle cure by the church, the International Medical Committee did not reach the two-thirds majority vote required to classify the case as unexplained.

When recounting this story, Dr. Theillier leans back in his chair and looks up. He has come to know Bély over the years, and the connection between doctor and patient is clear. His knowledge of the medical details is suffused with caring, with a sense of amazement at the cure, and with his own deep, abiding faith. When asked what it is about this place that could be helping patients to heal, the doctor again leans back and considers. He responds with the authority of someone who has lived with the question every day.

First of all, he says, there are the universal symbols—water, rocks, mountains—plus the grotto and the beauty of the spot. And of course there's the long history of the miracles. More important, Lourdes has a spirit of openness, an acceptance of being ill and of seeking and extending help, that can be felt by everyone who comes to the town. Underlying the entire experience is the profound faith that the visitors express and celebrate. They are bathed not only in the waters of the spring, but also in a chain of love and caring that extends back one hundred and fifty years. Cures may not be complete, says Dr. Theillier, but virtually every patient who visits Lourdes leaves feeling better, and most return year after year.

Jean-Pierre Bély was not the only patient with multiple sclerosis to be cured in a sudden and overwhelming state of ecstasy. Another, described in detail by Théodore Mangiapan in his book *Les Guérisons de Lourdes,* was the case of a Swiss Benedictine monk named Léo Schwager, who was cured of the illness in 1952 at the age of twenty-eight. For five years he had suffered recurrent episodes that included dizziness and speech impairment. Schwager finally came to Lourdes in April 1952, after a stroke left him paralyzed on one side of his body and unable to speak.

On the second day of his pilgrimage, when the procession carrying the Host was drawing near to him, Schwager stood up in a sort of ecstasy, then fell to his knees beside his wheelchair. "Suddenly I felt a shock, like electricity, and I immediately left my wheelchair, without even realizing what was happening to me. I found myself on my knees, following the Blessed Sacrament with my eyes until the procession was over, deep in my prayers." A physician who was nearby noted: "He had an air of extraordinary ecstasy. His gaze was fixed on the Blessed Sacrament as it moved away from him. . . . I noticed at the same time that he seemed physically shaken, as if he had been punched or struck with a violent emotion and had trouble taking a deep breath."

As soon as the service was over, Schwager realized that all his ailments had vanished: standing, walking, speech, vision, and appetite were all recovered in an instant. He returned to his monastery and to a fully active life. For forty years afterward he never missed his annual visit to Lourdes, where he became a brancardier, helping other pilgrims in their search for a cure. Unlike the case of Jean-Pierre Bély, Brother Schwager's case was certified as having no medical explanation, not only by the Lourdes Medical Bureau but also by the International Committee. In December 1960 the bishop of Lausanne, Geneva, and Fribourg declared his case a miraculous cure.

Many other pilgrims have described an overwhelming sense of love and warmth as the very first sign of a cure. A thirty-six-year-old woman, likewise suffering from severe multiple sclerosis, was diagnosed with the disease in 1996 and cured at Lourdes on May 20, 2004. Her testimony reads: "The first miracle of Lourdes, in my opinion, is the feeling you have when you enter the sanctuary—the sensation of entering a bubble of sweet gentleness and peace. The place is bathed in prayer, and the atmosphere is intensely warm with love. It is absolutely magical."

In a recent manuscript surveying patients whose cures were deemed miraculous, Dr. Bernard François, professor emeritus at the Université Claude Bernard in Lyon, reports: "In fifty-seven out of seventy-one cases, the clinical cure was instantaneous and perceived as an inner warmth, pains, an electric shock, a fainting spell, an invigoration, relief, and well-being. A state of ecstasy was observed by several physicians. Most importantly, the subjects exhibited a steadfast confidence that they had been cured."

There could be many reasons for such unexplained cures, especially cures that occurred more than a century ago. Diagnoses were less accurate. Some cases of multiple sclerosis or arthritis, for example, might have been caused by infections such as Lyme disease, which eventually cleared up. Still, the timing of the cures, which all coincided with powerful emotional experiences, points to the role of emotion in the healing process.

What is happening in the brain at such moments of intense emotion? Could it be that events in the brain have a healing effect on the bodies of these pilgrims? Just as when we are stressed the brain fires up its stress response, when we believe, it shifts into a *belief response*. It has taken researchers much longer to work out the biology of belief than to work out the biology of stress. Part of the reason is that it is easy to place an animal or a person in a stressful situation and measure something—a brain response, a hormonal response, a heart or immune system response. It's a lot harder to tell a person to believe, and then measure an effect. And it is impossible to do this in animals. In order to investigate the biology of belief in healing, scientists needed imaging technologies that allowed them to study the human brain at work. They also needed technologies that allowed unobtrusive measurement of changes in stress and immune responses. Even so, how do you know that a person is actually believing in something at the moment you choose to measure these outcomes? You don't. Research on the biology of belief had to be broken down into its smallest measurable bits, and until very recently this was impossible. Scientists who attempted such measurements were scoffed at and marginalized by their academic peers.

One of the most famous of these researchers was a French surgeon named Alexis Carrel. In 1912, he won the Nobel Prize in Medicine for research he had performed at the Rockefeller Institute for Medical Research in New York City. He had developed methods to grow cells in tissue culture outside the body, and surgical techniques to reconnect severed blood vessels. His work eventually made it possible to transplant whole organs, reconnect severed limbs, and reestablish circulation in the heart.

In May 1902, before Carrel performed his prize-winning research, he visited Lourdes. There he witnessed the cure of a young woman named Marie Bailly, who was close to death from tubercular peritonitis—an inflammation of the lining of the bowel and abdomen caused by the tuberculosis bacteria. This experience shook him to the core. He even wrote a semifictional account of it in a book called *The Voyage to Lourdes.* The book was not published until 1949, five years after his death, because his views had antagonized the French medical establishment. He had been forced to leave France and seek employment in North America, first at the Université de Montréal and then at Rockefeller University in New York, where he stayed until his return to France shortly before World War II. Despite his contributions to the field of medicine, Carrel died under a cloud: he was a supporter of the Nazi-allied Vichy regime. His reputation was forever tarnished, including his work on the miracle cures of Lourdes.

In *The Voyage to Lourdes,* he refers to himself as Dr. Lerrac— "Carrel" spelled backward. Far from being a dry academic account, the book explores his own gradual recognition that he was witnessing an unexplained phenomenon in which the body, through some incredible force attached to belief, heals itself more rapidly than can be explained by science.

In his detailed clinical descriptions of the miracle cures, Carrel observed that "the miracle is chiefly characterized by an extreme acceleration of the processes of organic repair." It is as if the body's healing processes undergo a fast-forwarding that seems to be precipitated by a state of prayer, profound belief, or ecstasy.

In today's world of space-age medicine, penetrated at every level by external cures—drugs, surgery, therapies of all sorts—we tend to forget that before the advent of antibiotics and surgical instruments, many people did survive all sorts of bodily insults: infection, trauma, childbirth, shock, and inflammation. Animals in the wild also survive without the benefits of medicine; they do it through their bodies' own healing mechanisms. The greatest miracle of all, as Carrel pointed out, is how this happens.

More than half a century after Carrel's death, technology had advanced to the point where researchers could begin to investigate how such cures might occur, and how belief could possibly promote healing. Although the mechanism of such cures is still not understood, many pieces of the puzzle have been solved. The organ that holds the answer is the brain.

In order to recognize and understand the brain's role in healing, scientists needed technologies that could monitor the brain at the moment people are feeling deep love, staunch faith, overwhelming joy, or profound tranquillity. They needed to know how such emotional responses could affect the immune system. Only then could they get an inkling of the possible biological basis for these cures.

The feeling described by the pilgrims at Lourdes during the first moments of their cures bears a remarkable resemblance in spirit, texture, and intensity to the feelings described by Buddhist monks who follow a type of Tibetan meditation called Loving-Kindness meditation, or *maitribhavana,* designed to achieve a state of great compassion, or *mahakaruna,* toward all living things. Much has been learned in recent years about changes in the brain during this kind of meditation, in large part due to a collaboration between Richie Davidson, a psychologist from the University of Wisconsin at Madison, and Tenzin Gyatso, the fourteenth incarnation of the Buddha, known universally as the Dalai Lama.

In 2005, the Dalai Lama made his first official visit to Washington, to speak at the Society for Neuroscience and the Mind and Life conference, a widely broadcast symposium on the neuroscience of meditation and the use of meditation in treating stress-related illnesses.

He had already conducted several such workshops at other sites, the first at MIT three years before. Each had consisted of two-and-a-half days of discussion-style panels bringing scientists and practitioners together to explore the science behind meditation and its potential health benefits. The workshops had grown out of his deep interest in science, particularly neuroscience.

The 2005 conference, entitled "The Science and Clinical Applications of Meditation," was conceived by a courageous group of neuroscientists led by Richie Davidson, who resisted attempts by the neuroscience community to distance itself from what was perceived as fringe science. Yet Davidson's research used the most advanced technologies available—fMRI and EEG technologies that were capable of measuring blood flow and electrical discharges throughout the brain and projecting them into 3-D images that could be mapped anatomically. Davidson had begun his work in this area within a network of scientists sponsored by the John D. and Catherine T. MacArthur Foundation. The MacArthur Foundation Networks were designed to foster research that was too creative, too novel, and too risky to be supported by government funds. Davidson's work fit all of those criteria perfectly.

His first project was a small pilot study of people who were learning to meditate. The CEO of a local biotech company wanted to encourage his employees to meditate and asked

Davidson for help in training them. Davidson saw this not only as an opportunity to help the company benefit its employees, but also as a way to study the effects of meditation on brain function and health. He divided the participants into two groups: those who were taught meditation, and a wait-list group who were given training brochures and pamphlets. He monitored the brain electrical activity of the meditation students using EEGs, and tested their immune system's ability to respond to a flu vaccine. He conducted the study in November, when the employees were receiving flu shots, so he was able to measure the blood levels of their antibody response to the vaccine. After only eight weeks of training, the participants showed increased electrical activity in the left prefrontal cortex—a region that is important in resilience and positive emotions. Davidson had previously shown that this area of the brain is more active in people who are resilient—those who have experienced major life crises from which they recovered with little or no long-lasting harm. At the same time, the meditators showed an enhanced response to the vaccine, an effect that was most marked in those who had experienced the greatest increase in brain activity. Yet despite the fact that the study was well designed and the findings tantalizing, the data from the trainees were, as Davidson put it, "all over the place." There seemed to be a trend, but no strong statistical significance. He suspected this might be because some trainees were better at meditating than others. What to do next?

Davidson turned to a long-standing relationship for the solution to his dilemma. In 1992 he had been invited to visit the Dalai Lama at his retreat in Dharamsala, India. The Dalai Lama had heard about his work on the neurobiology of emotions and resilience, and his previous studies on meditation, and wanted to learn more. He was even interested in neuroimaging his meditating monks. Davidson had visited Dharamsala, and so began a collaboration that had lasted for many years.

Now Davidson took his research problem to the experts, the Buddhist monks who were the Dalai Lama's followers— "the Olympic athletes of meditation," Davidson called them. He proposed a collaboration to measure the same brain parameters in meditating monks, and the Dalai Lama enthusiastically agreed. Davidson had the monks wear a cap embedded with 128 electrodes that could detect the brain's electrical activity while they meditated. The results of the study were published in 2004 in the *Proceedings of the National Academy of Sciences,* with an acknowledgment thanking "His Holiness the Dalai Lama for his encouragement and advice in the conducting of this research." The article received worldwide attention, not only in the scientific community but also in the popular press.

Several meetings at the Dalai Lama's headquarters in Dharamsala followed, bringing His Holiness and his followers together with neuroscientists. These gatherings were so successful that the conferences' sponsors, the Mind and Life Institute, decided to bring the experience to the rest of the world. The concept was to make people feel as if they were having discussions with the Dalai Lama in his living room. Except that the living room would be the stage, and the audience would have the opportunity to observe the discussions between the scientists and the expert meditators.

The Washington event of 2005 was fraught with controversy. The Mind and Life meeting was billed as an adjunct to the Society for Neuroscience conference. More than thirty thousand neuroscientists from around the world were expected to attend the main conference, where the Dalai Lama had been invited to give the keynote address, part of a yearly lecture series entitled "Science and Society" which examined the interface between science and important issues of the day—the same series at which Frank Gehry would speak the following year.

But several months before the November conference, a petition was signed by more than six hundred neuroscientists demanding that the president of the society withdraw the invitation to the Dalai Lama. It claimed that Davidson's 2004 paper was flawed, and that it had been funded by the Dalai Lama's supporters. News articles were written in scientific journals citing the petition's claims. The petition further stated that "the presentation of a religious symbol with a controversial political agenda may cause unnecessary controversies, unwanted press and significant divisions" within the Society for Neuroscience.

As reported by the *Washington Post,* "many of the petition signers were Chinese Americans, leading to countercharges that they opposed him [the Dalai Lama] on political grounds." The president of the society, Carole Barnes refused to yield to the pressure. "The Dalai Lama has maintained an ongoing dialogue with leading neuroscientists for more than fifteen years, which is the reason he was invited to speak," she said. So the Mind and Life conference and the keynote address to the Society for Neuroscience went forward as planned.

I was the moderator of the session on the use of meditation to treat stress-related illnesses. Prior to the session, I had been advised not to use the word "stress" in the discussions. The reason given was that stress was not a concept in the Buddhist tradition. The concept of anguish and suffering is embodied in the Tibetan word *dukkha,* but an equivalent for the word "stress" does not exist. But *dukkha* is akin to what we in the Western tradition recognize as depression, and depressive suffering is different from stress. Avoiding the word "stress" thus posed a serious dilemma for addressing the main topic of the session: whether meditation could be used to counter stress and the illnesses that stress might precipitate. How could we not use that word?

I decided to start the discussion by addressing the question head on. I said I understood that stress was not a concept in the Buddhist tradition, but that it would be difficult to have a discussion about the health benefits of meditation without address-ing this issue. I then asked the Dalai Lama, "Is there such a thing as stress in your tradition?"

The Dalai Lama turned to his translator. They conferred in whispers for what seemed like many minutes, seeking advice from another panel member, a translator and former Buddhist monk. There were more whispers back and forth. The 3,500 people in the audience waited.

Finally the Dalai Lama said, in English: "For the word 'stress' there is no proper translation." The translator revealed that they had been trying to find the closest term in Tibetan for the word "stress," but "His Holiness could find no equivalent term."

When I asked my next question, the floodgates opened: "This difference in the understanding of one word, 'stress,' cuts to the core of a very important difference between the two cul-tures, East and West. Since we in the West do try to use medita-tion to reduce stress, and since this is not a goal of meditation in your tradition, I would ask you to expand on what, in your view, its goal is in the Buddhist tradition."

The Dalai Lama's response was to outline the three main goals of meditation: cultivating ethical discipline, concentration, and insight. After expanding on each of the stages of the practice of meditation, His Holiness said, with a smile and a twinkle in his eye: "Universal compassion. That is all. Everything else, too complicated." The audience broke into applause and laughter.

So it seems that in one culture the goal of meditation is to en-hance positive emotions (love and compassion); in the other, it is to reduce negative emotions (stress and anxiety). Yet from a physiological point of view, enhancing the positive and reducing the negative will both ultimately improve health.

Throughout his entire visit to Washington, the Dalai Lama had been suffering from a terrible cold, coughing and sneezing through the day-long sessions. He began his keynote lecture by saying, in English, that in light of the controversy surrounding his visit, he would be reading his remarks—because he was feeling "unusual stress."

The next day, the *Washington Post* reported: "Because of the controversy over his speech to the neuroscientists in Washington, his aides said he would keep to a prepared text, something quite unusual for him. But he often diverged from the text, despite saying with a smile that he was feeling unusual 'stress.'" And John Geirland, in the online magazine *Wired,* wrote: "The fourteenth incarnation of the Living Buddha of Compassion approaches the podium, clears his throat, and blows his nose loudly. 'So now I am releasing my stress,' he says. The audience dissolves into laughter."

"The Living Buddha of Compassion" is a particularly appropriate name. The Dalai Lama practices what he preaches: in all his interactions, he expresses a deep and abiding compassion for others and for the world. The type of compassionate meditation that he and his followers practice is one of the oldest Buddhist meditative practices. It is a sitting meditation that involves slow, rhythmic breathing. Rather than emptying the mind, it requires active focus and nonjudgmental observation of the fullness of the mind. In order to achieve the state, the monks recite Buddhist tenets, or visualize the Buddha, or mentally articulate points in a debate justifying the importance of and strategies for achieving compassion. They may focus on an object of hatred or an enemy, in order to focus their mind on strategies to achieve tolerance for that object.

The word "compassion," derived from Middle English via Old French and ecclesiastical Latin, contains within it the word "passion." It comes from the Latin prefix *com-* ("with") and the verb *pati* ("to suffer"). Thus, it means "to suffer with," "to sympathize." *Pati* is also the root of the word "patience." The Dalai

Lama speaks to all these aspects of compassion when he describes the ways of attaining it. "To develop the practice of compassion to its fullest extent, one must practice patience," he says in his book *How to Practice: The Way to a Meaningful Life.* But more than this, "Real compassion is based on reason. Ordinary compassion or love is limited by desire or attachment."

As with breathing types of meditation, Loving-Kindness meditation affects heart-rate variability, altering heart rhythms from the adrenalin-like stress pattern toward the parasympathetic relaxation mode. When practitioners of this type of meditation achieve their perfect state of meditation—akin to achieving the "peak experience" called *kensho* or *satori* in Japanese Zen Buddhism—they experience what they describe as an overwhelming flood of positive emotions: warmth, love, peace, and compassion.

When Davidson measured electrical activity in the brain of meditating monks practicing this form of meditation, he made a startling discovery. What he had shown in his 2004 paper was that at precisely the point when the monks achieved their state of overflowing love and compassion, disparate brain regions, far apart and unconnected by any obvious nerve pathways, suddenly synchronized in a pattern of electrical activity called *gamma waves.* These are large waves that cycle at regular intervals. They are of a different frequency from the electrical waves that occur during sleep or waking. Those that characterize sleep are much slower, and those that characterize waking, the alpha waves, are much faster.

Though no one knows exactly what is happening in the brain during meditation, these changes are clearly associated with a particular mental state—one that is different from being awake and different from being asleep. It has a unique brain-activity signature. Some suggest that such synchrony is at the very root of consciousness, and that it plays a role in sustained focused attention. It may even be the basis of those "Aha!" moments that occur during learning.

When Davidson conducted functional brain-imaging studies of the monks, he found remarkable changes in brain blood flow, particularly in regions involved in love and attachment. These included areas that become active in both maternal and passionate love, as well as the regions that make up the brain's reward pathways—the same ones involved in addiction, sex, and music. Chief among the centers that became active was the nucleus accumbens (in the striatum), which controls desire. Other brain regions that lit up are involved in empathy, especially a region called the *insula*. According to Davidson, this area was brightest in the monks who experienced the deepest empathy and compassion.

It seems that monks who are highly trained in reaching this state can deliberately achieve it. Perhaps others who are not so trained can reach this state in other ways. It is not inconceivable that you could achieve such a sense of profound love and compassion by finding yourself in a place that inspires powerful life-altering belief, just as the pilgrims do at Lourdes.

What about prayer? Does the brain change when a person of deep faith is praying? Prayer is difficult to study, because a person can recite the words of a prayer, yet may not be in the state of ecstasy associated with profound belief. Just as Richie Davidson chose to study highly trained experts in meditation, namely Buddhist monks, other scientists have studied experts in prayer, including Franciscan and Carmelite nuns.

There are many ways to pray. One is to visualize the religious object, as Buddhist monks do. Another is to recite the words of a prayer. Andy Newberg, a neuroimager at the University of Pennsylvania in Philadelphia, conducted brain-imaging studies of Franciscan nuns while they performed a form of verbal meditation: repeating a phrase, as worshipers do when praying with a rosary. Newberg studied the nuns while they prayed. The type of brain imaging he used is called single-photon emission computed tomography (SPECT). The method relies on radioactive tracers to measure blood flow in different brain regions.

The nuns were asked to lie quietly in the scanner while they were injected intravenously with a radioactive compound whose radioactivity dissipates within minutes. An image of the radioactivity within the brain was collected, as a measure of their brain blood flow while they were at rest. The nuns then performed verbal meditation for fifty minutes, during which they were injected with another dose of radioactive tracer. They underwent a repeat brain scan half an hour later.

Newberg found that blood flow increased in several parts of the brain. He compared these scans to ones he had performed on meditating monks. Some of the areas that became active were the same that Richie Davidson had found, and some were different. The ones that differed were the ones related to words and vision. In the monks, the vision areas lit up but the word areas did not; in the nuns, the areas of the brain controlling words became active, while the vision areas remained quiet.

The areas that were similarly activated in the praying nuns and meditating monks were the reward circuits and the prefrontal and parietal lobes—those parts of the brain important in positive emotional responses and resilience. Clearly, the *way* the nuns and monks got to that emotional place mattered—whether through words or through vision. Once they reached that state of peace and love, the same brain regions became active: those that underpin passionate and compassionate love.

Sixty years after Alexis Carrel left the Université de Montréal, two researchers at that institution, Mario Beauregard and Vincent Paquette, using fMRI, performed brain-imaging studies on Carmelite nuns who had attained an ecstatic state through prayer. Many of the brain regions that became active in the Carmelites were those that became active in the Buddhist monks and the Franciscan nuns: those areas involved in love and compassion, as well as areas important in resilience.

All of these studies show that profound changes do occur in the brain during meditation and prayer—changes that create a unique state of mind different from wakefulness or sleep. It is a state that involves the parts of the brain that cause us to seek reward and feel joy when we achieve it. The pursuit of reward is even more powerfully felt than the achievement of it. In this pursuit, one must have an inkling of the possible reward that lies ahead. This inkling can be called hope, it can be called belief, or it can, in the most stripped-down scientific sense, be called expectation.

Whatever one believes about Bernadette's visions of the Virgin Mary—that the Virgin really did appear, or that Bernadette had some illness such as epilepsy or schizophrenia—one thing is certain. However you choose to interpret the miracle cures, there is no doubt that all who visit Lourdes leave the town feeling a little better and a little richer for the experience. Something very real happens at Lourdes, and it leaves no visitor untouched. There they find a loving, supportive community where people are accepted for who they are, no matter what their illness. And with them they bring their hopes and expectations for a cure. Two essential elements that can help an individual heal are expectation and social support. Lourdes offers both in massive doses.

How could this work? How do you get from a hope to a cure—from changes in the organ of emotions, the brain, to changes in the cells and organs of healing, the immune system? It took many teams of researchers expert in immunology, psychology, endrocrinology, and neuroscience six decades to figure this out.

9

HORMONES OF HOPE AND HEALING

When you feel better because you believe that something will heal you—whether that something is a drug, an action, a person, a procedure, or a place—you are experiencing the *placebo effect*. Unfortunately, this term carries a lot of baggage and is often preceded by the word "just," as in "just the placebo effect." People who feel better as the result of a placebo may be dismissed as gullible, hysterical, or malingering. Yet the belief that something has the capacity to heal is extremely powerful. Scientists must take it into account in every clinical trial designed to study the effects of a new drug or device before it is put on the market. Although the magnitude of the placebo effect is debated, researchers estimate that it accounts for at least 30 percent of the curative effect of any drug, and they must subtract this from the drug's total benefit in order to determine its "true" biological potency.

The type of illness being treated is important here, since different conditions respond differently to a placebo. Scar formation, say, is unlikely to be reversed by the power of belief. A placebo is likely to have a much greater effect on pain, which does not entail permanent physical changes; rather, it involves dramatic but more transient and more easily reversed chemical changes in nerves. As a result, some of the earliest and most clear-cut studies proving the biology of the placebo effect were performed with people experiencing pain.

In 1978, Jon Levine and Howard Fields at the University of

California in San Francisco were inspired by the then recent discovery that the brain had its own morphine-like molecules, called
endogenous opiates or *endorphins.* They used a drug that blocked
these molecules to figure out the chemical mechanism by which
placebo belief counteracts pain. The drug, called naloxone, has
no discernible clinical effect on its own; but when combined
with morphine, it completely blocks that analgesic's ability to relieve pain.

Fields and Levine chose a condition that was sure to be associated with pain: extraction of impacted wisdom teeth. The patients were told that they would be receiving morphine, or a
drug that might increase pain, or nothing at all. After the extraction, the patients were treated with morphine, or naloxone, or
a placebo—that is, an injection of sterile salt water (saline) that
contained no drug at all. Pain was reduced in the patients who
actually received morphine, and also in those who believed they
were receiving morphine but who received only saline. Even
more dramatically, the patients who received naloxone felt much
more pain than any of the other groups. The naloxone had
worsened the pain because it had blocked the effect of the
brain's own endorphins. These studies clearly showed that the
placebo effect has a biological basis that is at least in part due to
the brain's own opiate-like molecules.

Since the 1980s, when these studies were performed, scientists have developed new brain-imaging technologies that make
it possible to measure the release of nerve chemicals in different
regions of the brain. With these approaches, they can identify
the nerve chemicals that cause pain or relieve it. One of these
methods is positron emission tomography (PET scanning), the
same method that Marc Raichle used to visualize the brain's
tonotopic map. In this case, the high-energy radioactive tracer is
attached to drug-like molecules. The result is an image that
shows not only blood flow and metabolism in various brain re-

gions, but also the specific chemicals that are released in these regions when the nerve cells become active.

Jon-Kar Zubieta and his team at the University of Michigan in Ann Arbor performed PET studies using a radioactive tracer that attaches to opioid receptors in the brain. Zubieta gave healthy people a painful stimulus and then treated them with a placebo that they believed was an active painkiller. Their brain images showed that the greater the pain relief they experienced when given the placebo, the more of the brain's morphine-like molecules were released in those parts of the brain that control pain. This proved once again that the brain's own morphine-like molecules can be as effective in relieving pain as morphine itself, while avoiding the drug's terrible addictive side-effects. Besides activating opioid anti-pain pathways, the placebo stimulated other brain regions—the same areas that are activated by desire and by addictive drugs: the brain's reward pathways.

Just as there are many elements to stress and the response to it—the bad event, the physiological response, the perception that the event is bad—there are also many elements to the placebo effect, including passive expectation, conditioning, cultural factors, and social support. The first three are based on learning. In fact, expectation and conditioning are aspects of the same thing. Expectation is imperceptible learning that comes from everyday experience; conditioning is learning that comes from active training, the process of learning to associate one thing with another, as in Pavlov's dogs.

Expectation plays a very important role in the placebo effect. Fabrizio Benedetti, an elegant and charming Italian physician and neuroscientist from Turin, wanted to know how this worked. What are the brain's expectation pathways? He studied patients with Parkinson's disease, a condition that causes nerve cells to die in a part of the brain that governs movement.

Parkinson's patients gradually begin to experience muscle rigidity and difficulty initiating movements, such as rising from a chair or walking. It's as if their muscles were frozen or stuck, and in need of lubrication. Such patients must make an enormous effort to get going, and their movements are lurching and spasmodic. The same happens with their speech—it becomes slow and halting. They develop "rolling pill" tremors, which make them look as if they're rolling a pill between their thumb and forefinger. They may make other abnormal movements— jerks and twists seize them unexpectedly, as if they're being pushed by an invisible force. Eventually they are unable to move at all.

What is happening is that nerve cells are dying in a region of their brain important in controlling movement. Within this region lies another, the striatum, which is also part of the brain's reward circuitry. Nerve cells in this area produce dopamine—the nerve chemical that enables the reward-pathway cells to communicate. About 40 percent of Parkinson's patients experience depression, possibly related to the fact that they are missing this chemical of positive emotions.

The standard treatment for Parkinson's disease is L-Dopa, a chemical that nerve cells in this region need in order to make dopamine. In cases where L-Dopa fails, a new surgical technique has been developed that jump-starts these nerve cells with electrical stimulation. In this form of treatment, called *deep brain stimulation,* electrodes are implanted in the damaged part of the brain. Patients must be awake during the surgery, so that the surgeon can monitor the effects of the electrical stimulation and be sure that the electrode has been placed correctly. They feel no discomfort because the brain, though it controls sensation elsewhere in the body, does not itself sense pain.

In his studies of the placebo effect, Benedetti took advantage of the fact that he could not only ask patients how they felt and observe their movements during the surgery, but could also gauge the electrical activity of individual nerve cells by recording from the electrodes implanted in the brain. This allowed him to compare the effects of a Parkinson's drug with the effects of a placebo (saline).

The patients were all aware that they might be receiving either a drug or a placebo, but they didn't know which. Benedetti found that nerve-cell electrical activity decreased and movement improved in the patients who received the drug. The same happened in some patients who believed they were receiving the drug but who actually received the placebo. Those people who did not respond to the placebo showed no change in nerve-cell firing. So the expectation itself must have caused the release of nerve chemicals, which in turn altered the nerve-cell activity.

Raúl de la Fuente-Fernández and his colleagues at the University of British Columbia in Vancouver tackled the question of what those nerve chemicals might be. Fuente-Fernández was aware that under situations of extreme danger, patients with advanced Parkinson's are capable of movements they could not otherwise perform. Some are particularly susceptible to the placebo effect, and can, for short periods and with extreme effort, will their symptoms to improve. Fuente-Fernández postulated that in these circumstances the placebo might be causing the release of the patient's own dopamine (whatever small amounts remained).

He and his team performed PET scans on patients with Parkinson's disease. They used a radioactive tracer that binds to dopamine, and tested patients receiving a dopamine drug or placebo. The patients who received the drug all showed evidence of dopamine release in the affected brain regions. Among the patients who received the placebo, more dopamine was released in those who believed they were receiving the drug than those who thought they were not receiving the drug: the dopamine increased both in the part of the striatum that governs movement and in the part that governs expectation of reward. So once again, the expectation that something would heal was shown to release the brain's own nerve chemicals as effectively as a drug. In these studies, patients who received a placebo did not all show a benefit—clinically, electrically, or chemically. But the ones who did showed improvement in all those domains. Clearly, some people are more apt than others to respond to expectation with a full panoply of chemical and electrical brain responses; and when they do, the cure can be as effective as when achieved through a drug.

The pathways of belief and expectation thus include the endogenous opioid pathways, important in controlling pain, and the dopamine reward pathways, involved in addiction and desire. In the case of a placebo, it is the *expectation* of healing that triggers the reward cascade. The greater the expectation, the greater the quantity of nerve chemicals released, and the greater the nerve-cell activity in the brain's reward centers.

We all bring our unique set of expectations to every situation—whether it is the expectation that a pill will rid us of pain, that a prayer will heal us, or that a particular place will calm us. These expectations come from personal experience, general knowledge, culture, and history. Infants have no expectation that a medicine will heal. But as children grow, they become aware through personal experience and general knowledge that medicines can cure a fever, stop a cough, alleviate pain. The placebo effect is a big part of any healthcare professional's relationship with a patient, and is essential to the healing process.

Almost certainly it is this sort of expectation that pilgrims carry with them to Lourdes, and almost certainly such expectations contribute to the shrine's powerful effect on healing. Devout Catholics will know the legends of the miracle cures that took place at Lourdes; even before going there, they expect that visiting Lourdes and participating in its rituals will heal.

Whether it is one element of the place or all of its features combined that evoke such powerful emotional reactions is not known.

Some clues come from studies that test the association of a reward with preference for a place, the same type of studies that Linda Watkins and Steve Maier performed to test the effects of immune molecules on memory during illness. It turns out that both a single element of a space and the whole context have the ability to determine preference for place. In the first case, an animal can learn to associate a reward with each individual element of a space—say, the texture of the flooring. The magnitude of the effect is then equal to the sum of all the parts. In the second scenario, the entire context is associated with a reward, and all the elements combine to form a single representation of that environment in the animal's brain. It is the overall representation that gets associated with the reward.

Scientists need to do more work in order to understand how a particular place might heal humans. But these animal studies suggest that people who have learned to associate a place with a positive feeling—or with hopes that the place will heal—will benefit from simply being in that place.

Some of the beneficial effects of such places that promote healing might come in part from the same brain pathways that are activated during the placebo effect—the dopamine reward and opiate endorphin pathways. These positive emotional responses could trigger the release of nerve chemicals and brain hormones that stimulate the immune system to speed healing in the same way that worked in Pavlov's dogs: conditioning.

The first evidence that conditioning could affect the immune system came from studies performed in the 1980s by Bob Ader and Nick Cohen at the University of Rochester. Ader, a tall, imposing, confident man who bears a striking physical resemblance to Vladimir Lenin, is an authority in experimental psychology. Cohen is an immunologist—an expert in how immune cells function. With his long hair, beard, and sandals, he looks as if he would be more at home in a hippie commune than an ivory tower. When Ader and Cohen first reported their studies in the journal *Psychosomatic Medicine* in 1975, their claim—that one could train the immune system to respond to a conditioned stimulus, just the way Pavlov had trained his dogs—was widely challenged. Only after further studies, showing that they could condition many aspects of the immune response in different disease settings, were their findings finally accepted. The results were published in the journal *Science* in 1984.

Ader and Cohen studied mice that spontaneously develop systemic lupus erythematosus, an autoimmune disease that also occurs in humans. In this condition, the immune system attacks the body and causes inflammation in many organs, including the kidneys, lungs, heart, brain, and blood vessels. It even attacks the body's own blood cells. As the disease progresses, more and more antibodies are produced and more organs are affected; without treatment, the animal or human may die. The therapy involves drugs that suppress the immune system.

Ader and Cohen treated the lupus-prone mice with one such drug, called cyclophosphamide. As they predicted, antibody levels decreased and the mice lived. They then conditioned the mice to associate saccharin-sweetened water with cyclophosphamide. When the mice received only sweetened water after being trained to associate it with the immunosuppressive drug, antibody levels decreased and the health of the mice improved. Other mice received saccharin water without having been trained to associate the sweetener with the drug. These mice died.

The experiment showed that the immune system, like other physiological systems, could be trained to respond to conditioned or learned stimuli. This finding shocked most immunologists, who had assumed that the immune system didn't need the body to guide it. This assumption was based on the fact that immune cells function well in a culture dish, where they can grow, multiply, gobble up debris, make antibodies or immune molecules, and kill viruses or cancer cells. Scientists even doubted whether the immune system could be influenced by nerves, nerve chemicals, and hormones, let alone by something as vague as learning. But Ader and Cohen reasoned that if a dog can learn to associate a random stimulus like a bell with food, and salivate when it hears the bell alone, then a mouse could learn to associate the taste of sweetened water with an immunosuppressive drug and tune down its immune response. And if mice could do it, why not people? It took Ader and Cohen nearly a decade to persuade their peers that this reasoning was correct.

Today there is no question that the phenomenon is real. It has been replicated many times, most notably by Manfred Schedlowski and his team in Essen, Germany, who performed Ader and Cohen's experiments in people. They trained volunteers to associate a sweetened drink (green-colored strawberry milk flavored with a drop of lavender oil) with an immunosuppressive drug. When the researchers later gave the participants the drink together with identical-looking capsules containing no drug, they found that the participants' white blood cells made fewer immune molecules and grew less, just as if they had received the immunosuppressive drug.

How could a learned expectation in the brain affect the way immune cells fight disease? The German researchers tackled this question by giving the participants a drug that is usually used to treat high blood pressure and that blocks the adrenalin-like nerve chemical norepinephrine. They were able to prevent the placebo-induced immunosuppression with that drug, thus proving that part of the placebo effect is mediated through these adrenalin-like nerve chemicals. This provided a plausible mechanism for the effect of a placebo on immune-cell function, since others had shown many years before that such nerves course throughout the spleen, lymph nodes, and other immune organs where immune cells grow and mature. Virginia "Ginny" Sanders at the Ohio State University and Cobi Heijnen in the Netherlands provided the final link. Their work suggested that, during placebo expectation, it was these adrenalin-like nerve chemicals that were at least partly responsible for changing immune-cell function.

Another piece of the puzzle fell into place at the Mayo Clinic in Rochester, Minnesota, at once harking back to the miracle cures at Lourdes and changing the future of medicine.

As you drive south from Minneapolis and St. Paul toward Rochester, you pass fertile rolling hills planted with corn and soybeans. In the latter half of the nineteenth century, immigrants from Europe saw the potential of this rich black soil and moved here to escape scarcity in their native lands. The population grew, and with it the need for schools and doctors. In 1852 a country doctor named William Worrall Mayo arrived in St. Paul by steamboat from the East, joining the large community of Catholic settlers and missionaries. Dr. Mayo served as a Union surgeon during the Civil War, and afterward set up practice in Rochester with his sons Will and Charlie, also physicians.

In August 1883, a tornado destroyed one-third of Rochester. There was no hospital in the town. The injured were brought to hotels, a dance hall, and the Academy of Our Lady of Lourdes, a convent and secondary school founded by Catholic nuns, the Sisters of St. Francis of Our Lady of Lourdes. Mayo, his sons, and the Sisters joined forces to care for the victims. When the worst was over, the founder and head of the convent, Mother Alfred (born Maria Moes in Luxembourg), proposed an audacious plan to Dr. Mayo: she would raise money to build a hospital if he would promise to run it.

The hospital they built, St. Mary's, became renowned for its surgical successes. It combined the latest antiseptic techniques with the Sisters' devoted care. Its surgical suites were the most advanced in the nation. The large windows and skylights admitted abundant natural light; the floors were tiled and equipped with drains to allow easy application of antiseptic sprays. The hospital introduced an operating table, based on a Viennese design, that was state-of-the-art: a wooden trestle-table whose slats were covered with waterproof cushions and which had a tin trough underneath to catch body fluids and antiseptics. In fact, antiseptic was sprayed so liberally that patients and staff almost seemed to be showering in it.

Such innovations paid off. While overall hospital mortality rates at the end of the nineteenth century ranged around 25 percent, St. Mary's had a mortality rate of just 2 percent—close to miraculous in those days, when infection was rampant. The hospital and its parent organization, the Mayo Clinic, built a worldwide reputation for the very best surgical and medical care.

Even though the cures depended on advances in modern medicine, the Sisters played a very important role. Members of the Order of Saint Francis of Assisi, they followed that saint's tenets: live a simple life, promote education, minister to the poor, and help those unable to help themselves. But their more immediate inspiration was an event that had taken place just twenty years before Mother Alfred founded her convent: the miracle at Lourdes. These brave nuns, despite the odds, were able to create a healing place in frontier America which lasted and grew to what it is today. Rochester, with the Mayo Clinic as its core, is now a healing city to which, in an eerie parallel to the town of Lourdes, thousands flock from all over the globe. But instead of expecting miracles, the sick who come here pin their

hopes on the latest advances in medical science. One of the as-
tounding cures that contributed to the Mayo Clinic's fame occurred in 1948. The discovery provided another piece of the
puzzle for how hope can heal.

A twenty-four-year-old woman named Mrs. Gardner developed
stiffness and pain in her hands. She had trouble opening jars and
buttoning her coat. Her finger joints swelled and she began to
drop things. Her knees, wrists, and shoulders began to ache. She
felt as if she had a case of flu that never cleared.

Her doctor took X-rays and ran some blood tests, and diagnosed rheumatoid arthritis. He prescribed aspirin, but even
massive doses had little effect. Mrs. Gardner began to notice de-
formities in her fingers and wrists. Her fingers were stuck in a
flexed position; her knees and ankles began to swell; her toes became deformed, like her fingers. She took to her bed, exhausted,
depressed, and losing weight.

After four-and-a-half years of illness, Mrs. Gardner was admitted to the Mayo Clinic, where a rheumatologist named
Philip Hench was testing new treatments. She was hospitalized
for two months while several different injections were tried, but
none worked. The pain and weakness were so severe that she
could hardly get out of bed, but she refused to be discharged
until a treatment could be found.

Dr. Hench had noticed some years before that his patients
with rheumatoid arthritis, who were mostly female, experienced
relief of symptoms when they became pregnant or if they developed jaundice. He was convinced that a substance released by
the body during pregnancy or jaundice—he called it Substance X—would help to cure this illness. Over the years he had
tried treating his patients with several hormones, including female sex hormones, but none seemed to have an effect.

His colleague Dr. Edward Kendall, head of the Mayo's Department of Biochemistry, had been working since 1935 on isolating and preparing compounds extracted from the adrenal glands of cattle. He had already discovered thyroid hormone (from thyroid glands) and adrenalin (from the core of the adrenals). In May 1948, Kendall and his colleagues at the drug company Merck created a new preparation, which they called Compound E and which was extracted from the adrenal cortex (the outer casing of the adrenals). It was tested in patients with Addison's disease—an illness in which the adrenal glands fail. These patients suffered from profound weakness and fatigue; the drug restored their strength. Hench immediately applied to Merck to try it in his rheumatoid patients, in part because they experienced the same kind of weakness and fatigue that the Addison's patients had.

On September 21, 1948, Dr. Hench's assistant, Dr. Charles Slocum, injected the first dose of Compound E into Mrs. Gardner's arm. On the second day of treatment she found that her joint and muscle stiffness were abating. She also felt a sense of euphoria and well-being that she hadn't known in years. Her appetite returned. After just four daily doses of the drug, her condition had improved so markedly that she was able to walk out of the hospital unaided.

What was this miracle cure? Its chemical name was 17-hydroxy-11-dehydrocorticosterone. It has since become widely known as cortisone. Hench tested it on fifteen more patients with rheumatoid arthritis, and in April 1949 he published his results in the *Proceedings of the Staff Meetings of the Mayo Clinic*. In 1950 he published the results of a larger study in which twenty-three patients were treated with cortisone, some in conjunction with the pituitary hormone ACTH. Twenty-two of these twenty-three patients experienced marked improvement. Joint and muscle stiffness decreased dramatically within two days of the first injections. Joint pain, tenderness, and swelling decreased after eight days and markedly improved within two to three weeks. In 1950 the Nobel Prize was awarded to Hench, Kendall, and Tadeus Reichstein, the Swiss chemist who had identified the chemical structures of several hormones related to cortisone. Many people believe that Hans Selye also deserved to share in the prize, for his monumental work in compiling knowledge of the steroid hormones and their structure. It is indeed odd that none of the Nobel acceptance speeches acknowledged Selye's contribution.

Today, cortisone is used with rapid results in many preparations. Whether rubbed on the skin, inhaled in a nasal spray, injected into joints, muscles, or veins, or taken by mouth, it quickly resolves the pain and swelling of inflammation. It was one of the first great miracle cures of the twentieth century, and is still one of the most potent anti-inflammatory drugs available.

The way cortisone works may shed light on the miracle cures experienced at Lourdes. The body's own cortisone, the hormone cortisol, is produced by the adrenal glands not only during stress, as Selye had predicted, but also during any powerful emotional experience. The cortisol released from the adrenals is as potent an anti-inflammatory drug as cortisone, and keeps the immune system in check, preventing it from attacking the body. When the immune system is conditioned, as in Ader and Cohen's experiments, the placebo association keeps it in check through hormonal responses like the release of cortisol, as well as through those adrenalin-like nerve routes that Schedlowski had discovered.

When healing takes place without any apparent external cause, it may be because these kinds of hormones and nerve chemicals are released in the brain and body. A powerful experience, such as the ones that occur at Lourdes, could stimulate massive activation of the dopamine reward pathways or opioid pain pathways in the brain, which in turn could trigger a massive release of the anti-inflammatory hormone cortisol into the bloodstream. At the same time, adrenalin-like nerve chemicals could be released into the spleen and other immune organs. If this were the case, these hormones and nerve chemicals could have profound and rapid effects on alleviating pain, lifting mood, facilitating movement, and reducing inflammation.

But cortisol is not the only healing hormone released during such emotional experiences. The patients who were cured at Lourdes also described overwhelming feelings of love and peace. Are there beneficial nerve chemicals or brain hormones released at these moments of profound compassion?

Nearly a century after Alexis Carrel carried out his Nobel Prize–winning work at the Rockefeller University, another Rockefeller scientist named Donald Pfaff traced the regions in the brain that control passion-like behaviors in mice and hamsters. For many years, Pfaff had been studying the nerve routes and brain chemicals that control a graceful movement seen in female rats and mice—indeed most mammals, including cats—when they are in heat. Stroke a cat slowly from the nape of her neck down to her tail and you will see a slow and sensual arching of the back, ending with the rump exposed and raised. This movement, called *lordosis,* is a reflex, but one that female mammals of many species perform when ready to receive the male. It also enhances sexual desire in human females during intercourse. What Pfaff discovered is that the lordotic movements of the female mouse, and those of the male when he mounts her, are driven by areas in the brain that govern desire, and their matching hormones that control all aspects of reproduction.

The hormones that choreograph these behaviors are *estrogen,* which regulates ovulation in females, and *testosterone,* which controls spermatogenesis in males. Yet another hormone, a small almost-protein or peptide called *gonadotropin-releasing hormone* (GnRH), must also be released in the brain of both the female and the male for the entire process to occur. Moreover, these same hormones are needed for the male to seek out and communicate with the female during mating. He does so in a series of approach behaviors that are mediated first through odor, then through sound, and finally through touch.

When hamsters begin their mating ritual, the male leaves a signal that is diffuse in time and space and depends on his testosterone. His scent, or "mark," is released from sebaceous glands on his flanks, but he can produce it only if he is able to make testosterone. In response, the female releases a "mark" of estrogen-dependent secretions from her vagina, leaving a trail behind her as she slinks into her burrow. The male then follows her, now emitting a signal that is diffuse in space but not time— ultrasonic vocalizations. She in turn emits ultrasonic calls from her hiding place. He follows both her scent and vocalizations, to find her and enter the burrow. From then on, all is touch. Now, even the gentlest stimulation of her skin will send her into full lordosis.

In Pfaff's words, these experiments proved early twentieth-century physiologist Walter B. Cannon's classic concept of "the unity of the body": the same hormones needed for fertility orchestrate the behaviors that allow the male and female to mate. This unity linking brain pathways of desire to sex hormones' control of reproductive organs has striking parallels in the way brain pathways of reward, desire, and belief are activated in the healing process.

The brain regions that become active during the mating sequence include those that are part of the brain's reward system. Besides being important in mating and sexual behavior, these regions are important in pair bonding and attachment associated with maternal behavior: the ultimate universal form of compassionate, altruistic love.

Just as the male and female sex hormones, and the master hormone in the brain which triggers their release, orchestrate a set of behaviors essential to mating, so do hormones released by the brain orchestrate behaviors needed by the pair once they have reproduced. These behaviors—maternal behavior toward offspring, pair-bonding between mother and offspring, and bonding between female and male—together constitute the biological essence of attachment and compassionate love. Like the sex hormones, the hormones of attachment control not only behavior but physiological responses needed to produce and raise the young. They are the hormones of parturition (childbirth) and of milk letdown. They are also active in the male and female during sexual excitement, desire, and successful completion of intercourse. They also have a powerful effect on the immune system and the way it helps the body to heal.

In the late 1980s and early 1990s, a small group of researchers in Maryland, just outside Washington, D.C., were trying to identify the brain chemicals involved in affiliative behaviors and pair-bonding. Sue Carter, a petite woman with long curly blonde hair, was a scientist in the Department of Zoology at the University of Maryland at College Park. For many years, she had been studying the social and mating behaviors of a small mouse-like creature called a prairie vole. Tom Insel, a psychiatrist (and Gene Kelly look-alike) at the National Institute of Mental Health, was studying brain pathways of a hormone called oxytocin, important in milk letdown and childbirth. Insel and Carter soon pooled their resources and began studying the problem of the role of the brain hormones oxytocin and vasopressin in social and affiliative behaviors and pair-bonding. The animals they chose to study were the voles, whose social and mating behaviors Carter had already characterized in detail while she was an assistant professor at the University of Illinois at Urbana-Champaign.

The area around Urbana-Champaign is largely rural farmland—the heart of the midwestern Corn Belt, whose black, deep, loamy soil supports mainly corn and wheat. It is a perfect natural habitat for the prairie vole, which likes tall prairie grasses, unlike its cousin, the montane vole, which likes mountain regions. In part because of habitat and scarcity of food, the social structure of the prairie vole evolved to favor monogamy, strong pair-bonding between male and female, and two-parent care of the young. In contrast, montane voles are not monogamous. The males show low levels of social attachment, and do not contribute to parenting.

Carter's studies of voles had focused on the hormone oxytocin, which is released during nursing and childbirth in all mammalian species. It causes smooth muscle to contract, precipitating uterine contractions during childbirth and milk letdown in nursing mothers. It is produced in the hypothalamus—the region of the brain that controls the stress response—but it is made in the posterior portion of this region, rather than in the anterior half, where the stress hormone CRH is made. It is then secreted from nerve endings into the pituitary gland just beneath the hypothalamus, where it is stored until a stimulus comes along to trigger its release.

There are many such stimuli: childbirth, nipple stimulation during nursing, the sex hormones estrogen and progesterone. Activities involved in sexual behavior, including genital stimulation, will also trigger oxytocin release in both the male and the female. The trigger can be learned through conditioning, so that actual tactile stimulation may not be necessary to cause its release; a memory or an association recalling the tactile stimulus may be sufficient. A classic example of this is the milk letdown that occurs in nursing mothers when they hear an infant's cry. The oxytocin that is released during nursing increases pair-bonding between mother and offspring. When released during copulation, it increases attachment to the mate.

Before beginning his collaborations with Sue Carter, Tom Insel had mapped the brain distribution of receptors for oxytocin. He had found that these molecules, to which the hormone must bind before producing its effects, were elevated in the brains of female rats immediately after the birth of their offspring. Many researchers, including Carter, had proposed that oxytocin might play a role in the contrasting social behaviors and pair-bonding in the different types of voles. Insel took the next logical step: he studied the expression and distribution of oxytocin receptors in the brains of prairie voles and montane voles.

Insel did find contrasting patterns of expression for receptors of oxytocin in the monogamous prairie voles compared to the polygamous montane voles. The monogamous males had more receptors for oxytocin in parts of the brain governing attachment, while the polygamous males had fewer receptors. Insel published his findings in the *Proceedings of the National Academy of Sciences* in 1992; he proposed that the binding of this hormone to its receptors in emotional centers in the brain may play a role in the pair-bonding that accompanies mating, nursing, and childbirth. Carter and Insel went on to study the voles' brain distribution of vasopressin, a hormone that is released from the pituitary gland at the same time as oxytocin and which causes aggressive behaviors in males. Once again they found differences in levels of this hormone in the monogamous and polygamous voles. They published their findings in the journal *Nature* in 1993. These papers became the foundation for a comprehensive theory of the role that these brain hormones play in various aspects of love: sexual, affiliative, and maternal. They even play a role in trust and generosity.

At every stage, from desire to mating to raising offspring, the brain and the body are flooded with a range of hormones that influence behavior and mood: the sex hormones estrogen and progesterone, the lactation and parturition hormones oxytocin and vasopressin, and another lactation hormone called prolactin.

What does all this have to do with healing? It turns out that each of these hormones has profound effects on the immune response, in some cases enhancing and in others suppressing inflammation and the ability of immune cells to fight infection. Their precise effect on immunity depends on the particular hormone, the type of immune cell, and the timing and amount of the hormone that is released. But that they do affect immunity is beyond doubt. Estrogen enhances immune cells' ability to recognize and respond to foreign invaders, and strengthens inflammation. Females of all species, whether mouse, rat or human, have a twofold to tenfold higher incidence of inflammatory diseases like arthritis, in part because of this effect. In contrast, progesterone, like cortisol, tunes down the immune response. This may be why pregnant females of all species are more prone than males to certain infections: the female body produces large amounts of progesterone, especially toward the end of pregnancy. Prolactin tunes up the immune response, and is elevated in certain autoimmune diseases like lupus. Drugs that block prolactin can even reverse or slow symptoms of lupus in mice that develop the disease spontaneously.

The pair-bonding hormone oxytocin affects the immune system in two ways. By tuning down the stress response, it helps to buffer the negative effects of stress. Both oxytocin and its receptors are also expressed in cells in the thymus gland's immune nursery, where new immune cells are "educated" to tolerate immune triggers called antigens. This prevents the immune system from attacking the body. Researchers at the Ohio State University tied together these various effects of oxytocin and demonstrated their importance in wound healing, which depends on a fully intact immune system. In a study of Siberian hamsters, a species that pair-bonds like prairie voles, they showed that social isolation prolongs wound healing by increasing the stress hormone cortisol; pair-housing the animals protects them from this effect. Treating the hamsters with oxytocin sped wound-healing, while treatment with a drug that blocked oxytocin significantly increased wound size and slowed healing.

If all these hormones affect the immune system, is there any evidence that positive emotions can improve health in people? In fact, there is. Richie Davidson, and now scientists at Emory University, have found that compassion meditation improves immune function. Compassionate and altruistic activities are also associated with better health outcomes in the people practicing them. Many studies, particularly in the elderly, have shown that those who volunteer have longer life spans and better mental and physical health. It may be that healthier people are the ones who volunteer in the first place. But one group of researchers in Marin County, outside San Francisco, found that elderly volunteers had health outcomes over a five-year period that were 63 percent better than those of people who did not volunteer, even when controlling for factors such as illness, which might prevent volunteering. Other studies have shown that people with many social ties and social interactions have better health outcomes, fewer emergency room visits, and fewer and less severe upper-respiratory infections, such as flu or the common cold.

In cases such as the cures of Jean-Pierre Bély and Léo Schwager at Lourdes, or of the thirty-six-year-old woman who recovered miraculously from multiple sclerosis, all these factors might have come into play: compassion, passion, ecstasy, and the accompanying activation of brain pathways and release of hormones that could heal. One difficulty in proving the cause of sudden cures from diseases like multiple sclerosis is that such autoimmune diseases often wax and wane on their own. Sometimes they flare up, then enter a period of quiescence that may last months or years, then resume again. It could be that internal factors such as the natural waxing and waning of hormones might enhance and greatly speed the body's own healing processes. Research has certainly shown that stress can trigger or worsen the disease. Why couldn't the opposite—profound compassion and ecstasy, and the hormones that are released during these states—help to alleviate or change the course of illness?

If there *were* a biological explanation for the resolution of these patients' symptoms, it would not diminish the wonder of the phenomenon. The miracle is that faith can be so profound and powerful that it could help to trigger the internal healing pathways of the brain and body.

If places like Lourdes can mobilize the body's own healing processes, why not incorporate some of their elements into hospitals? In fact, architects and healthcare design professionals are beginning to do just that.

10

HOSPITALS AND WELL-BEING

Roger Ulrich, buoyed by the evidence he gathered in his 1984 study showing that windows with views of nature speed healing, devoted the rest of his career to applying these principles to healthcare design. If he could scientifically identify the features that gave window views their healing powers, perhaps he could provide architects and designers with the ammunition they needed to convince clients to build hospitals in a way that optimizes healing. He set about systematically studying each element that could account for the outcome of his study. Was the crucial factor nature itself? Could artwork or images have the same effect? Was the factor light? Sound? At the same time, he began advising architects and designers on ways they could design hospitals that incorporated these principles.

Out of these efforts grew a field called *evidence-based design*. It uses physiological and health-outcome measures—length of stay, amount of pain medication, complication rates, and patient stress, mood, and satisfaction indices—to evaluate the health benefits of architectural features in hospitals. Many projects around the country are gathering evidence to determine whether such design innovations will benefit patients, their families, and hospital staff, and whether they will reduce healthcare costs by speeding recovery and reducing complications and medical error rates. The collaborators in these projects include healthcare architects, environmental psychologists, government agencies, private foundations, manufacturers, and hospital administrators, all of whom see an advantage to incorporating these new design principles into hospitals.

In June 2004, at the request of the Robert Wood Johnson Foundation, a nonprofit organization engaged in healthcare research funding, Ulrich and health psychologist Craig Zimring, a professor at the Georgia Institute of Technology in Atlanta, presented their work at a panel convened at the National Press Club in Washington, D.C. Their findings did indeed attract media coverage, so novel was the concept of designing hospitals to maximize healing!

The gathering was small, by invitation only, but most of the major players were present, including healthcare architects and designers, manufacturers, and members of the Agency for Healthcare Research and Quality (AHRQ), the U.S. government body that funds research in healthcare quality and delivery. Also present were two representatives from the Academy of Neuroscience for Architecture (ANFA), whose goals and mission began where Ulrich's work left off. I was one of those representatives. ANFA's stated purpose was less practical: to discover the neuroscience underlying the effects of built space on thought processes, memory, and mood. But the two domains, theoretical and applied, had reached a comfortable and collegial working relationship.

It had become apparent that a major source of complications in patients are the features of hospitals that increase the likelihood of healthcare provider errors. The Institute of Medicine had outlined these findings in a 1999 report entitled *To Err Is Human*. The report had received massive press coverage, followed by public and congressional outrage at the current state of affairs in U.S. hospitals. The report asserted that as many as 98,000 Americans die every year in hospitals as a result of preventable medical errors—more than from motor vehicle accidents, breast cancer, or AIDS. Anything that could be done to counter the situation would benefit patients, healthcare providers, and institutions.

The Clinton administration had responded quickly. It issued an executive order instructing government agencies that dealt with healthcare programs to implement proven techniques for reducing medical errors, and it created a task force to find new ways of reducing errors. Congress launched a series of hearings on patient safety, and in December 2000 it allocated $50 million for AHRQ, to support efforts aimed at error reduction.

The report listed hospital design as one important area to be targeted:

> The AHRQ already has made major progress in developing and implementing an action plan. Efforts under way include:
>
> - Supporting new and established multidisciplinary teams of researchers and health-care facilities and organizations, located in geographically diverse locations, that will further determine the causes of medical errors and develop new knowledge that will aid the work of the demonstration projects.
> - Supporting projects aimed at achieving a better understanding of how the environment in which care is provided affects the ability of providers to improve safety.

This was precisely the goal of evidence-based design, and the report and the subsequent infusion of funds did a great deal to advance the field. At the Robert Wood Johnson workshop, Ulrich and Zimring presented their most recent work, in which they had reviewed more than three hundred evidence-based design studies to assess effects on hospital care. Outcomes fell into three main categories: patient safety, environmental stressors, and ecological health. Factors that improved safety included reduced infections, reduced injuries from falls, and reduced medical errors. Factors that contributed to environmental stress included noise in the hospital environment. Features that increased comfort and support for patients and staff, such as visitor areas and green spaces, fell into the category of ecological health. The results of the survey were so impressive that AHRQ used it as the centerpiece for a 2005 white paper assessing the status of the field and setting future funding priorities.

Ulrich reported that one of the biggest stressors in a hospital environment is noise. A number of studies have shown that hospital noise generally exceeds the recommended level of thirty-five decibels (a quiet office), and usually falls in the range of forty-five decibels (room conversation) to sixty-eight decibels (loud music heard through headphones). But levels can go even higher.

In 2004, at St. Mary's Hospital of the Mayo Clinic, nurses placed hidden noise gauges in the Surgical Thoracic Intermediate-Care Unit. They found that decibel levels were especially high when staff were changing shifts and when heavy equipment such as portable X-ray machines was being moved around. Sometimes noise levels reached ninety-eight decibels—as loud as a motorcycle.

Many studies have shown that noise in this range increases heart rate, blood pressure, and other measures of stress. It certainly interferes with sleep—another physiological function necessary for healing and psychological well-being. Studies performed in some children's hospital intensive-care units showed that such noise levels not only interfere with falling asleep and staying asleep, but also result in poor sleep quality.

In an attempt to evaluate potential beneficial effects of structural corrections in acoustics, researchers in a Swedish hospital replaced sound-reflecting ceiling tiles with sound-absorbing tiles in a coronary intensive-care unit. They found, not surprisingly, that the noise levels were substantially reduced. Not only did health outcomes improve, with fewer rehospitalizations, but the staff's satisfaction and home sleep quality improved as well.

The reason for all this noise lies in the long history of hospitals, which originally were not places where people went to heal, but places where people went to die. Until the early twentieth century, the vast majority of patients who entered the hospital exited through the morgue, because they died from infections they had acquired while in the hospital. So people rightly tried to avoid hospitals as much as possible. Then healthcare professionals realized that the design and contents of hospitals, and the building-influenced behaviors of the doctors and nurses in them, were the source of those infections. In their eagerness to rid hospitals of infection, architects and designers of the twentieth century removed all possible elements that could spread infection, including any sort of surface that could harbor germs. The only way to keep these places clean was to cover them with metal, stone, or tile—materials that were acoustically reflective. As hospitals became cleaner, they became colder, noisier, and less comforting. "Sterile" became a negative term.

A sterile room is one stripped bare of ornament and color, with shiny metal surfaces, tile on the floor, no plants or accumulations of personal objects—a room that is pristine, germ-free, and easy to keep clean. This was a good thing—even a breakthrough in modern hospital design, when the main concern was risk of infection. Of course minimizing risk of infection is still a major issue in hospital design, but it is a given, a necessary starting point. What patients now crave is more attention to their states of mind and emotions, and to all those things in the environment that sustain them.

The evolution of hospital design from ancient times has paralleled the course of infectious diseases and the knowledge of germ theory that helped to prevent and cure them. The ancient Greeks and Romans did not have hospitals as we know them. Greek medicine was divided into two streams. One was the Hippocratic movement, in which itinerant doctors moved from

town to town, treating the ill in their own homes, using principles that are still the basis of clinical medicine today: the history
and the physical. Through careful questioning and palpation of
the body, the doctor could identify clues about the nature and
course of the illness. The better a doctor was at detecting subtle
signs of an illness, the better he would be at predicting the outcome, and as a result, the more patients would flock to his care.
The Hippocratic branch of medicine was founded on this sort of
diagnostic acumen.

In the other, parallel system, patients who were considered
chronically or terminally ill visited temples to the Greek god of
healing, Asclepius, for their care. These temples were built far
from the heat, noise, dirt, and dust of the towns, always at freshwater sources, usually with a magnificent view of the sea. Patients were treated with healthy diet, pure water, music, sleep
and dreams, social interactions, and above all prayer.

Ancient Rome had no hospitals either. Soldiers were treated
on the battlefield. Lepers were segregated in colonies, not for
their own benefit but for the protection of society, to prevent
the spread of the disease.

The first hospitals as we know them were built by knights
of the Middle Ages: the Templars, and the knights of the Order
of St. John of Malta. These sanctuaries were meant to help trav-
elers along the various trails to holy sites—the routes of Cru-
saders to the Holy Land and those of pilgrims to Santiago de
Compostela. The only building in Santiago that matches the cathedral in size and grandeur is the Hostal de los Reyes Católicos,
or Royal Hospital. It was built by King Ferdinand and Queen
Isabella in 1453 to express gratitude for the independence of
Spain from the Moors and to care for the pilgrims who streamed
into the town. It is now a luxury hotel. Its huge vaulted ceilings,
spacious hallways, and quiet courtyard lined by a wide colon-
nade all testify to the vast crowds of sick who passed through its

wrought-iron gates. It is thought to be the oldest hospital in the Western world, built expressly to care for the sick.

Other hospitals, often attached to a church, were located all along the Camino Frances that ended at Compostela. There were also tiny hospices, where pilgrims could rest for the night and seek assistance for their ills. The smallest of these were stone huts with dirt floors, often built in the cool forest shade next to a refreshing stream. They were among the first local hospitals or clinics. Today many have been transformed into hostels where modern pilgrims who hike the trail can rest overnight for a minimal fee. Arriving at one after a ten-kilometer trek in the 100-degree summer heat is truly a soothing relief.

As in developing countries today, the major diseases that plagued the world centuries ago were infectious diseases: infections in wounds sustained on farms, in kitchens, and on battlefields; infections contracted during childbirth; infections spread from person to person in dirty, crowded environments. The most dire was of course the Plague itself, the Black Death, which killed millions throughout the Middle Ages. Although the existence of germs was known since 1683, when Anton van Leeuwenhoek had first viewed the tiny "animalcules" through his microscope, their role in causing infections was not recognized until centuries later.

In the nineteenth century the fever that resulted from infections during childbirth, called *puerperal fever,* was rampant in hospitals. As a result, women feared hospitals, and childbirth almost always took place at home, supervised by midwives. It was not known that the major source of these infections was the doctors themselves, who would go directly from the autopsy table of one patient to the delivery table of another without changing their coat, washing their hands, or wearing gloves.

In 1843, the American physician Oliver Wendell Holmes, and in 1849 the Hungarian physician Ignaz Philipp Semmelweis, independently proposed that thorough hand-washing could prevent puerperal fever in childbirth. Both were ostracized by their medical colleagues as a result. Holmes presented his recommendations in a report to the Boston Society for Medical Improvement and published them in an obscure journal. They were derided as unnecessary and went unheeded. Semmelweis, an assistant lecturer at the Vienna Lying-In Hospital, encountered similar resistance. He had noticed that women admitted for childbirth to the hospital's two wards had very different rates of puerperal fever. He performed a study that was effectively what today is called a *randomized controlled clinical trial*—and was able to do this because, as it happened, women were randomly admitted to the two wards on alternating days. Semmelweis found that mortality rates were much higher on the first ward than on the second: 16 percent, as compared to 7 percent. He noted that women admitted to the second ward were exclusively cared for by midwives, while those on the first ward were cared for by doctors who went directly from the autopsy room to the delivery room. Semmelweis instituted a rule that doctors scrub their hands with a weak chlorine solution before attending a delivery, and the infection and mortality rates on the first ward dropped to match those on the second. Though his colleagues derided his observations and he lost his position at the hospital, his ideas found acceptance in the late 1850s, toward the end of his life. Hand-scrubbing with disinfectant is still one of the most effective ways to prevent the spread of infection.

By the late 1800s, French chemist Louis Pasteur was convinced that germs caused disease. He discovered a way to protect animals and people from infection by injecting them with germs that had been killed by heat. Pasteur prevented anthrax infection in sheep in this way, and also sterilized milk by heating it, a method called *pasteurization* which is still used today. Then he saved the life of a boy who had been bitten by a rabid dog.

The seemingly miraculous effect of the injection he adminis-tered—the first rabies vaccine in history—finally convinced his colleagues that his theories were correct.

The foundation of germ theory was fully articulated by Ger-man physician Robert Koch, who in 1882 discovered the bacte-ria that cause tuberculosis and cholera. He developed a set of rules which are the cornerstone of modern microbiology. Ac-cording to these rules, called *Koch's postulates,* simply finding a germ in a person with a certain illness is not enough to prove that the germ caused the disease. Experiments must be done ex-posing animals to the germs in question, and only if a similar ill-ness develops in the animals can one conclude that the particular germ is the cause of the disease. It was the solidification of this theory—of cause and effect between exposure to germs and the diseases that result—which convinced the medical community that microscopic germs do indeed cause infection.

If germs spread infections, then one important way to pre-vent and cure infection should be to kill those germs or clean them away before they have a chance to take root in the patients' tissues. It was Scottish surgeon Joseph Lister who put these ideas into practice. A surgeon at the University of Glasgow, Lis-ter knew of Semmelweis' work and Pasteur's germ theory. He based his recommendations for antiseptic techniques in part on Pasteur's ideas and in part on his own observations. In 1867 he published his recommendations in the *Lancet* and the *British Medical Journal,* with a preamble saluting Pasteur: "When it had been shown by the researches of Pasteur that the septic property of the atmosphere depended on . . . minute organisms suspended in it, . . . it occurred to me that decomposition in the injured part might be avoided by applying as a dressing some material capable of destroying the life of the floating parti-cles." He proposed that all surgical instruments and the pa-tients' wounds be doused in a weak solution of carbolic acid to make the entire surgical area "anti-septic." This innovation was adopted around the world and resulted in greatly reduced infection-related mortality. It was these procedures that the Mayo Clinic employed so successfully in the late nineteenth and early twentieth centuries. They form the basis of the antiseptic techniques used today: surgeons scrub their hands with antiseptic soaps, change into sterile gowns, sterilize their instruments, and use antiseptic solutions to clean the area of the incision.

The design of hospitals changed to accommodate these advances in knowledge. One of the greatest proponents of hospital reform was Florence Nightingale. During the Crimean War of 1854–1856, British soldiers wounded in battle on Russia's Crimean Peninsula were ferried across the Black Sea to the barracks hospital in Scutari, Turkey. Conditions there were abominable, and mortality rates were as high as 60 percent. Patients were left to fester in their own excretions, bed sheets were covered with excrement and blood, wards were so crowded that lice migrated from bed to bed, and the rooms were dark and airless. Nightingale, a vigorous leader and superb organizer, changed all this. She and her team of nurses washed the soldiers' bodies with clean cloths, boiled the sheets, made sure the beds were spaced well apart, let sunlight and fresh air into the wards, and prepared nourishing, easily digested food for the patients. Hospital deaths declined dramatically.

In England after the war, Nightingale became a vocal advocate for hospital reform. She was a proponent of the ideas of British architect Henry Currey, who designed London's St. Thomas Hospital in 1868. This landmark opposite the Houses of Parliament was built on the *pavilion principle*, which emphasized ventilation, airiness, and sunlight. The design originated in post-revolutionary France, and was based on a plan by architect Bernard Poyet. Each pavilion was provided with rows of large windows and with long hallways, which allowed for cross-ventilation. The sanitary facilities were located far away from the patients. Beds were spaced well apart and were placed near the window bays.

These principles of hospital design soon spread throughout the world. The mid-nineteenth century records of the Montreal General Hospital contain handwritten notes of the hospital's board meetings. The budget of one report in the 1860s requested funding for hospital improvements—items such as wooden sidewalks leading to the outhouses, to protect patients' feet from mud in rainy weather. The Royal Victoria Hospital, also in Montreal, was built in 1893 and looks like a turreted gray-stone Scottish castle—not surprisingly, as it was designed by British architect Henry Saxon Snell to resemble one, at the request of its Scottish-born financiers. It grew by accretions over a century, and each new wing reflected the latest advances in hospital design. By the end of the First World War, the Royal Vic boasted many features considered state-of-the-art. In the public wing and the maternity wards, enormous windows and twelve-foot ceilings let in air and sunlight. The nursing stations were centrally placed so that the head nurse had a clear view of all her patients—sometimes as many as thirty to a ward. Curtains could be drawn between the beds for privacy. In the 1930s a wing was added for wealthier patients, with light-filled rooms containing only one or two beds. Each new wing was built in a terraced fashion, cut into the hillside and the woods, so that—in keeping with the Modernist movement of the time—patients were provided with access to nature. This was especially true of the nearby Children's Hospital, where nurses wheeled their young charges out in day beds or let them play in gardens so they could take the air.

The Royal Vic also kept the autopsy area separate from the hospital. The pathology building, constructed in 1923, was safely located across the street. To get there, the gurney and its shroud-covered load would be wheeled into a large cage elevator. The operator would shut the heavy metal gate and the body would descend to the basement where it was wheeled along a subterranean passageway. In the 1970s you could visit this underground route, which seemed to take you back to the nineteenth century. Offshoots of the corridor led to a honeycomb of dimly lit, low-ceilinged rooms with musty earthen floors, gray stone walls, and wooden trestle-tables here and there. Whatever one imagined went on in those rooms (carpentry? laundry? autopsies?), it was well away from the patients.

These advances, which seem so primitive now, revolutionized the way patients were cared for. They led to impressive declines in infection rates and altered the public's perception of hospitals as death traps. But they also led to the barrenness and stressfulness of today's hospitals. Shiny, easily cleaned surfaces reflect and amplify sound. The trend toward single rooms to limit the spread of infection increased patients' isolation. Limitations on visits from family and friends, again to minimize infection, contributed even more to isolation. The increasing emphasis on diagnosis and diagnostic equipment meant that hospitals were devoting more and more space to machines rather than to people and healing.

As hospitals grew to accommodate these new technologies, so did the paths that patients had to take as they made their way through the buildings. Navigation through a strange and often frightening environment, harboring unfamiliar instruments lurking in intimidating procedure rooms, is an extremely stressful and anxiety-provoking experience, especially for someone who is ill and already primed for fear. Add to this the blurred memory, impaired cognition, and depressed mood that immune molecules cause during illness, and stress and distress increase even more.

Research has shown that stress is harmful to health. It slows healing, predisposes the body to more severe and more frequent infections, and compounds the effects of illness. A hospital environment, whose goal is to heal, should do what it can to eliminate stress.

Jan Kiecolt-Glaser and Ron Glaser at the Ohio State University in Columbus were among the first to prove the effects of all kinds of stressors on the immune system, particularly on wound healing and on the immune-cell functions that protect against infection. They began their research in the 1980s, when the merging of a "soft" science like psychology with a "hard" science like immunology was still frowned upon by their more biologically oriented colleagues.

Kiecolt-Glaser is a petite woman with a blond pageboy and blue eyes. She speaks in measured tones, and usually ends her sentences with a warm smile. A clinical research psychologist who trained at the University of Miami and the University of Rochester, she became interested in the effects of stress on health—unsurprisingly, since both schools were known for their research in health psychology. The University of Rochester was home to the psychologists George Engel and Franz Reichsman, who in the 1950s had done seminal work on the effects of isolation on physiological responses, and also home to Bob Ader and Nick Cohen, who had proved that immune responses could be linked to a psychological stimulus via conditioning.

Glaser, a tall, imposing man, was trained in virology and immunology and was a self-proclaimed skeptic of the softer sciences. His research at Ohio State involved isolating and growing viruses, and isolating different types of immune cells in order to study how they kill viruses. This was something you could see under a microscope; it was not something vague, like emotions or stress.

But Glaser wanted to find a topic on which he and his wife

could collaborate. He was casting about for a subject when his father died and he found himself in a period of grieving. A physician friend told him that he'd better watch his health, since some research showed that people going through a period of mourning were more susceptible to illness. He found his topic: the Glasers decided to study immune responses during bereavement.

Their first experiments indeed showed that the immune response in widowed spouses of Alzheimer's patients was impaired. In particular, immune cells known as *natural killer cells,* which are critical in fighting viral infection and killing cancer cells, were weakened. The Glasers extended their research to wound healing in women who were caregivers of Alzheimer's patients. They cut tiny biopsies, the size of pencil erasers, from the skin of volunteers, and measured the time needed for the wounds to heal in stressed and nonstressed individuals. They found that the wounds in the caregivers took about ten days longer to heal than those in women of comparable age and income who were not under chronic stress. They also examined the possible influence of stress on the effectiveness of vaccines. They gave flu shots to medical students undergoing exam stress, and measured the amount of antibodies that were produced in the blood. When the students received the vaccines during a stressful period before exams, vaccine effectiveness was lower and the students made fewer antibodies than they did when the vaccine was administered during a vacation period. Finally the Glasers measured the effects of marital stress on the functioning of immune cells in the blood. They asked couples to choose a subject that was a bone of contention (money or in-laws, for example), then collected blood and measured the couples' immune-cell function before, during, and after the argument. They found that immune functioning was impaired, especially in the women whose style of argument involved confronting their husbands and whose husbands' style of argument was to withdraw. Jan

Kiecolt-Glaser admits that it is these studies on marital discord and its deleterious effects on health which seem to resonate most with people.

Another psychologist-immunologist research team, Sheldon Cohen and Bruce Rabin at Carnegie Mellon University in Pittsburgh, studied the effects of chronic stress on severity of infection with the common-cold virus. Using questionnaires, they measured stress levels in 349 volunteers and then exposed them to measured amounts of five different cold viruses. They quarantined the volunteers and waited to see if they developed a cold. The higher the stress levels people reported before the exposure, the more likely they were to get sick and the more severe their illness.

In all of these cases, stress clearly impaired the ability of immune cells to fight infection and promote healing. Comparable results were obtained in studies of a variety of other stressors. Physical stress, such as rigorous exercise, impairs immune-cell function and weakens resistance to infection. Lack of sleep over prolonged periods elevates stress hormones, depresses immune-cell function, and reduces the effectiveness of vaccines.

Something that's just as harmful to health as stress is isolation. In the 1950s, George Engel and Franz Reichsman proved that isolation and environmental deprivation were associated with physiological changes. They studied a one-year-old infant named Monica who was born with a gastric fistula—a hole that connected her stomach with the outside of her abdomen. While she was in the hospital waiting to undergo surgery to correct the defect, she was kept in a metal crib covered with pristine white sheets and was given little visual stimulation. She was left alone for many hours while the nurses went about their daily routine with other patients. Engel and Reichsman noticed that she exhibited signs of depression: fear, withdrawal, crying, and loss of appetite. When her favorite nurse entered the room, she perked up and smiled and cooed. They then measured the volume of the gastric secretions that flowed from the fistula, and found that when Monica was depressed and sullen and withdrawn, these slowed to barely a trickle. When she was happy, the juices started flowing again.

Indeed, positive social interactions are important buffers against stress. Sheldon Cohen and Bruce Rabin found that the more types of social interactions people reported over a period of time, the fewer upper-respiratory infections they developed. Cohen and Rabin concluded that the social support derived from these interactions helped to ward off infection.

Patients in the hospital are constantly exposed to stressors that impair health, slow healing, and weaken the immune system. Understanding and reducing stress in the hospital environment is to twenty-first-century medical care what understanding germ theory and reducing infection were to nineteenth-century care. Advances in psychology and neuroscience now provide a scientific basis for taking into account the effects of emotions on disease. This knowledge can do for hospital design and health-care today what germ theory did in the nineteenth century. A precursor of this notion was common in nineteenth-century hospital design, but like everything else in the medicine of that era, which separated the mind and the body, features of the physical environment which supported a healthy mind were applied only to hospitals for the mentally ill.

St. Elizabeths Hospital, just outside Washington, D.C., was built on land purchased by the federal government in 1852 at the urging of the social reformer Dorothea Lynde Dix. Dix was on a mission to develop a nationwide system of charitable institutions to care for the mentally ill, at a time when such care was largely nonexistent. St. Elizabeths was to be the flagship hospital in a more enlightened era of caring for the insane. Dix had as her ally the prominent physician Charles Henry Nichols, who was appointed the hospital's first superintendent even before construction began. This permitted him to help design the building, modeled according to the plans of his mentor, Dr. Thomas Story Kirkbride, who served as superintendent of the Pennsylvania Hospital for the Insane from 1841 to 1883.

The site for St. Elizabeths was chosen by Dix and Nichols. They had three criteria in mind, consistent with Kirkbride's recommendations. The location had to be out in the country; it also needed to be close enough to the city for easy access to amenities, especially railroads and a water supply; and it needed to have sweeping vistas.

Saint Elizabeth of Hungary is the patron saint of hospitals and nursing homes, but this is not the reason for the hospital's name. As a federal facility (the first of its kind) in a country that mandates the separation of church and state, the facility could not be named after a religious figure. It was originally called the Government Hospital for the Insane. Yet it was built on land that, in the seventeenth century, had been known as the "St. Elizabeths tract." And this epithet, complete with its archaic disregard of the apostrophe, survived. An act of Congress made the name "St. Elizabeths Hospital" official in 1916.

A ten-foot wall of brick and stone completely encircles the campus. When you come through the gates, you see a three-story redbrick building in front of you and the skeletons of greenhouses off to your right. The overall atmosphere is one of peace and calm. Traffic noise has given way to birdsong. A wide, grass-covered alley flanked by white oaks leads to the main building. Here is where the wealthy families of the mentally ill would arrive on horse and buggy, passing between the rows of stately oaks.

Nichols selected Thomas Ustick Walters as his architect—a brilliant choice that would ensure the creation of an imposing

structure, just as Nichols and Dix wanted. Walters was the architect of the Capitol and its dome, which was under construction
in the years 1855–1866, at the same time the hospital was being
built. The main building looks like a redbrick fortress, complete
with turrets and battlements on top. The linear layout incorporates four staggered wings off a five-story central tower. Each
wing is lower than its neighbor, with the tallest ones closest to
the tower, a stepped design that ensures ample light and airflow.

Kirkbride's principles of design for moral treatment of the
insane came to be known as the Kirkbride Plan, and influenced
the design of virtually all American mental institutions in the
late nineteenth and early twentieth centuries. They grew out
of the early nineteenth-century asylum movement in England
and France. They held that a hospital's physical features had to
support emotional and mental health by providing spaces for
physical activity and beautiful surroundings. Scattering gardens,
fountains, and summerhouses throughout the grounds not only
camouflaged the hospital's custodial nature, but created a place
for patients to enjoy, a rural haven where their emotions could
be soothed. Though many of Kirkbride's other principles and
those of his peers are anathema in our era, his theories were
based on humanitarian ideals at a time when more effective therapies for mental illness did not exist. They also stemmed from
his own experience. Kirkbride had grown up on a farm. A
Quaker, he was convinced that the hard work and daily exercise
of farm life were essential to mental health. He wanted a place
where patients could move about freely; where they could socialize and take their meals together in a community; where they
could read, play games, and work the land. And he believed in
beauty. In his 1854 treatise *On the Construction, Organization
and General Arrangements of Hospitals for the Insane,* he wrote:
"The surrounding scenery should be of varied and attractive

kind and the neighborhood should possess numerous objects of an agreeable and interesting character."

The soil had to be easily tilled, so that patients and staff could work side-by-side on the farm and in the gardens to produce food for their meals. The hospital building had to be situated so as to assure views from every window, especially from the parlors and rooms where patients congregated during the day. Flowers were to be grown in greenhouses, and picked daily to decorate the halls and common areas of the hospital. According to the *Pennsylvania Hospital Newsletter of the Friends of the Hospital,* "Dr. Kirkbride . . . believed that the beautiful setting . . . restored patients to a more natural balance of the senses."

Situated along the bluffs overlooking the confluence of the Potomac and Anacostia rivers, St. Elizabeths, now a National Historic Monument, has all this in spades. It sits on the rim of a topographic bowl in which Washington, D.C., is located. On the opposite edge of the bowl, at one of the highest points in Washington, sits the National Cathedral. Between the two, easily visible in a grand vista from a spot known simply as the Point, are many of the city's greatest landmarks: the U.S. Capitol, the dome of the Library of Congress, the Old Post Office Building, the Jefferson Memorial, the Washington Monument, the Old Executive Office Building, the Pentagon, Reagan National Airport, Bolling Air Force Base, the Naval Research Labs, and the Coast Guard Headquarters. So close is St. Elizabeths to these important facilities that today the grounds are off-limits to the public, in part for security reasons.

The hospital's buildings, some of them uninhabitable, now sport peeling paint, leaky roofs, and rusty pipes. The site's overseer is not a psychiatrist (the last of those retired in 1987) but an asset manager for the U.S. General Services Administration, the agency that maintains many of the federal buildings across the country. Familiar with every inch of the place, he and the GSA ensure that the buildings are kept in reasonable repair, and work with government agencies that might occupy and restore the structures to their former glory. The Department of Homeland Security is now slated for the site.

Nowadays, most of the few hundred psychiatric patients at St. Elizabeths are treated on an outpatient basis. One of its most famous residents was John Hinckley Jr., who attempted to assassinate President Reagan in 1981. Another famous inmate was the poet Ezra Pound, who lived and worked there from 1945 to 1958. Pound was vilified for making anti-Semitic, pro-Fascist radio broadcasts from Italy during World War II. Upon returning to U.S. soil, he was arrested for treason, but the court declared him insane and he was committed to St. Elizabeths. His room, like all the others, was tiny—eight feet by ten feet—and had a window reaching two-thirds of the way to the fifteen-foot ceiling. Opposite the window was an equally tall door with a transom, to capture the summer breezes off the river and allow warm air to circulate from the state-of-the-art heating system.

The asset manager, looking like a construction worker in boots, jeans, and a shirt with rolled-up sleeves, but with jacket in hand, took me on a tour of the place. As we entered the main hospital, a musty smell enveloped us; I stepped hesitantly onto the uneven floorboards. From there, we went through darkened hallways, under wide arches, to a room directly below the one that Pound had occupied. It was tiny—no bigger than a monk's cell in a monastery. But, as my guide explained, the patients were not meant to stay in their rooms. They only slept there, spending their waking hours out on the grounds or in the common areas, most of which had windows with spectacular views. Pound read voraciously, translated Sophocles and Confucius, received visitors such as T. S. Eliot, and completed two volumes of his *Pisan Cantos*. He also played daily tennis games with the staff on the clay courts outside his room. But life was not easy for Pound and his fellow patients, who were liable to be subjected to the primitive treatments of the day.

As we wandered through the long-disused spaces, I was struck by the decrepit grandeur of the redbrick buildings—close to seventy of them on that vast bucolic campus. I imagined the busyness and the hum as patients worked the fields, which sloped toward the river above the old Civil War cemetery. They harvested corn, baked bread, raised vegetables, grew flowers, tended fruit trees. In contrast, at the back of the hospital, several buildings were spaced around a wide lawn shaded by holly trees, blossoming magnolias, and white oaks. It resembled a college quadrangle or town green, with a fountain at its center, surrounded by a fire station, creamery, bakery, upholsterer, and library. St. Elizabeths was not only a working farm. It was, as my guide put it, a "completely self-sustained village," and it thrived over the decades.

Unfortunately, Kirkbride's idealistic theories could not withstand Victorian-era pressure to control the mentally ill and hide them from society. The grounds and buildings may have been designed for humane care in an idyllic setting, but the methods used to treat the patients back then were often harsh, with straitjackets and other forms of torturous physical restraints and punishments. The reputation of such institutions suffered, and asylums were replaced by more modern approaches to mental-health care.

Yet Kirkbride's basic doctrine still holds: hospital spaces should be designed to support the emotions and lift the spirits. This principle should apply not only to facilities that treat mental illness, but to all healthcare institutions. We need to merge this principle of mental support, and the role that place can play in it, with the advances that have taken place over the past century in medicine for the body. We need to bring the mind back into the equation of health and healing, and include the ways that emotions and the physical environment interact, for the benefit of patients with both physical and mental ailments.

A knowledge of how built space can affect moods and physiological responses, and how those in turn can affect the health of patients and staff, could provide the evidence and motivation for funding the construction of spaces that foster emotional and physical health. Resistance to implementing such advances today stems not only from ignorance and entrenched dogmas, as it did in the nineteenth century, but also from the high cost of building and technology. The best way to counter this resistance is through research that can furnish persuasive data—proof that changes in hospital design which reduce stressors can also speed healing, and will therefore benefit both the health of patients and the hospital's bottom line.

This was precisely the goal of the 2004 Robert Wood Johnson Workshop in Washington. It was also the goal of a workshop organized by the Academy of Neuroscience for Architecture at Woods Hole in 2005. This particular workshop aimed to take some of the principles already discussed and apply them to the analysis of architectural plans. It brought together architects, neuroscientists, and environmental psychologists for a brain-storming session. The neuroscientists with expertise in stress looked at architectural drawings of various hospital units. With large felt pens, they marked features that could exacerbate stress: narrow hallways, rooms near noisy nursing stations, lack of privacy for families, windows with dispiriting views, and so on. Then the architects proposed possible solutions. The session gave everyone an appreciation of the importance of scientific principles, and how easily they could be applied to real-life settings to improve patient comfort and health.

Besides removing stressors from the environment, healthcare

design research aims at adding features that enhance comfort and take into account the spiritual and social aspects of the patient's life. This is what Roger Ulrich has referred to as *ecological health*. It includes the addition of gardens, views of nature, artwork, soothing music, nature sounds, soothing colors, and spaces where family members can congregate for mutual support. This category also includes environmentally friendly or "green" features, such as construction materials that improve indoor air quality by reducing noxious gas, renewable energy systems, recycled water for irrigation, open spaces, nature trails, balconies, and gardens. A branch of architecture called *biophilic design* takes this one step further: it espouses the notion that nature itself has a healing effect. This idea is not so far from the Modernists' belief that incorporating nature into housing and hospital design can improve health.

A spectacular example of this type of hospital design is the Mayo Clinic's Leslie and Susan Gonda Building, which opened in 2001—a tribute to the medical advances of the twenty-first century that has won numerous design awards. Its remarkable features begin with the lobby, a three-story atrium of glass, marble, and steel designed by Ellerbe Becket and Cesar Pelli and Associates. Hanging from the ceiling are brightly colored blown-glass chandeliers by the artist Dale Chihuly. These sculptures, reminiscent of sea-spray or something that might have been churned up on a windswept beach, diffuse the light and draw your eye upward. On the walls are huge paintings and murals by contemporary artists, some quite well known. The atrium also contains gentle auditory stimulation; the soothing sounds of a grand piano fill the space. Anyone is welcome to play here, and many musicians come to volunteer their time. An enormous window—an entire wall—overlooks a terraced rock garden that's planted all year round, even in winter, when it sports purple ornamental cabbage. Seats along the glass wall face toward the garden. Patients and family members congregate there—some standing, some sitting, others pushed in wheelchairs by relatives or nurses. None are facing toward the interior of the building; all are gazing out at the terraces bathed in bright sunlight. The overall effect is one of peace and tranquillity, even though the space is large and usually filled with dozens of people hurrying by.

Such innovations in hospital design are being applied at facilities across the country, and current research is assessing their health benefits in order to determine which aspects of design work and which don't. One of the difficulties with this sort of research, which tests the effects of built space on health outcomes, is that constructing a building is not a trivial task. It's impossible to build an ideal hospital as an experiment simply to measure its effects on health. How does one address this challenge?

A group of architects, environmental psychologists, and leaders in healthcare design conceived of a way to do this. The collaboration was initiated by a not-for-profit organization in California called the Center for Health Design. The results were presented at the 2004 Robert Wood Johnson Workshop.

The team realized that the best way to gather data on new aspects of design would be to study many small projects rather than design a single big hospital. They hoped that the results of each small study would have ripple effects, like so many pebbles thrown into a pond. Hence the name of their collaboration: the Pebbles Project. Each subproject dealt with a different kind of hospital or unit: hospitals for children, for rehabilitation, for long-term care; units for intensive care, cancer therapy, and cardiac treatment. Each obtained stringent measures of health outcomes, and gathered input from patients, family members, and staff. The Pebbles Project involved hospitals located all over the country, from San Diego and Palo Alto in California, to St. Paul,

Minnesota, and Indianapolis, Indiana, to Kalamazoo and Detroit in Michigan, all the way to Derby, Connecticut.

At Methodist Hospital in Indianapolis, the staff noticed that frequent transfer of patients from high-level cardiac intensive care to the step-down unit was extremely costly and a source of medical errors. The solution the design team proposed was to enlarge the rooms, so that a patient could stay in the same room when being shifted to intermediate care. Half of each large room contains the hospital bed and all the equipment and supplies needed for cardiac emergencies. The other half looks more like a living room, with comfortable chairs, side tables, plants, a sunny window, and artwork on the walls. This arrangement reduces the risk of errors, since it allows the same staff members to take care of the patients throughout their hospital stay. It also gives family members a pleasant place to sit, thus enhancing the social support that is so important in healing. This simple change resulted in a 90 percent decrease in transports, 75 percent fewer falls by patients, and greater patient and family satisfaction.

The Barbara Ann Karmanos Cancer Institute in Detroit remodeled one of its units with soothing colors and comfortable furniture, and added Internet access outside every patient room for staff, patients, and family members. The designers also reorganized supplies, increased the size of medication rooms, and installed acoustic tile in the ceilings. They then compared health outcomes in the new unit with those on an existing old unit. They found that on the new unit, patients used 16 percent less pain medication and errors decreased by 30 percent.

At Bronson Hospital in Kalamazoo, where several alterations were made, including strategically placed sinks, hospital-acquired infections fell by 11 percent. Comparable benefits were evident at San Diego Children's Hospital after it provided its medical and surgical units with access to balconies and garden views.

One could go down the entire list of Pebbles sites, and in every case improvements were clearly associated with better health outcomes. Not only that, but they saved money and made hospitals better places to stay in, to work in, and to visit.

In 2003, Derek Parker, a principal at the healthcare architecture firm Anshen and Allen in San Francisco and a founder of the Center for Health Design, was searching for a way to present the findings of the Pebbles Project in terms that would resonate with healthcare design professionals and hard-nosed industry leaders, whose bottom line was the bottom line. He hit upon an idea: he would combine the data from the project's many small successes into a total picture of what a hospital could be. Parker came up with an imaginary state-of-the-art facility that he called the "Fable Hospital," whose design, health outcomes, and costs were based on the real numbers derived from the individual units in the Pebbles Project. The results, which he published in the journal *Frontiers of Health Services Management* in 2004, made the business case for such design innovations. The Fable Hospital included oversized single rooms to reduce transfers, minimize infection, and increase social support; "acuity adaptable" rooms, where patients requiring different levels of care could be continuously housed; double-width bathroom doors, allowing caregiver and patient to enter side-by-side; decentralized nursing stations; air filtration; hand-sanitizer dispensers near every bed; peaceful settings; bigger windows; noise-reduction measures; patient-education centers; and staff-support facilities. By Parker's calculations, the enhancements would cost $12 million, but nearly the entire amount—a total of $11 million—would be recouped in the first year. What's good for the health of patients and staff seems to be good for the hospital's bottom line as well.

What is the future of healthcare design? Are there organizations that are developing these principles? At least two furniture

manufacturers are deeply committed to improving hospital design for patients, family, and staff. They work closely with the
Center for Health Design, the Pebbles Project, and many other
healthcare research and funding organizations. Both are located
in Grand Rapids, Michigan, and both have a long history of development and innovation in furniture manufacture.

In the town of Holland, Michigan, on a point of land jutting
into Lake Macatawa, sits a Prairie Style stucco and wood-trimmed
lodge named Marigold. The original owner, Egbert Gold, was
an inventor from Chicago whose family had made a fortune at
the turn of the twentieth century designing residential heating
systems. He commissioned a student of Frank Lloyd Wright to
design a summer home for his wife, Margaret. The many windows, framed in Wright-style stained glass, give onto views of
the lake and the property, landscaped with shade trees and wil-
lows. The winding road to the lodge takes you through woods
of tall trees, so tall that you have to crane your neck out the car
window to see the lowest branches. Arriving here at night, you
might easily feel like Dorothy setting out on the Yellow Brick
Road. Indeed, it was close to here, on the other side of Lake
Macatawa, that Frank Baum wrote *The Wizard of Oz* in 1900.

This is western Michigan forestland. Dutch settlers came here
in the late 1800s because of the trees. They were fine-furniture
craftsmen who sought the tall, straight pines and oak for their
trade. Their legacy is apparent not only in the displays of tulips
every spring, but also in the area's many Dutch names, including that of their town. By the mid-twentieth century the fine-
furniture industry had moved to the Carolinas. But another
type of furniture manufacture took its place, one that combined
new materials such as steel and acrylic with traditional ones like
wood, cane, and leather. Its pieces had sleek modern lines, and it
now catered to the world of business.

Two companies based in Grand Rapids, Steelcase and Herman Miller, are leaders in both office furniture and healthcare design. Steelcase was founded by the Wege family in 1912, and made its mark patenting fireproof steel waste-baskets, filing cabinets, and desks. Herman Miller was founded by Dirk Jan De Pree and named for his father-in-law, whose loan helped to start the company in 1905.

Herman Miller now owns the Marigold estate, and uses it as a learning center. When you enter the lodge, you're surprised to see that the furniture is much more contemporary than the lodge. The Modernist chairs are immediately recognizable as the signature molded-plywood loungers and chairs of Charles and Ray Eames, the husband-and-wife team who designed for Herman Miller in the 1950s and 1960s. These chairs, created (in the Eameses' words) to "fit like a baseball glove," actually do: they curve to the small of the back and support it. They were designed with people in mind.

The idea of creating chairs out of a single piece of molded plywood had been around since the early 1930s, but the technology was not available to manufacture them. The plywood refused to bend in more than one direction without splintering. For years, the Eameses tried to find a method for producing molded plywood reliably, cheaply, and quickly. The breakthrough came from an unlikely source: the battlefields of World War II. In the early stages of the war, the U.S. Medical Corps had a problem. The metal splints that were placed on wounded soldiers being carried off the field were causing more harm than makeshift wooden ones, because the metal amplified vibrations, whereas wood dulled them. The Eameses worked with the military to develop molded-plywood splints that were lightweight and comfortable. They were given access to classified information about new synthetic glues and plywood production processes, and after the war they were able to use these processes to manufacture their trademark chairs. In 1946 Herman Miller began to market the Eameses' chair designs. This was perhaps the first time that design merged with healthcare advances to form people-friendly products that were ergonomically shaped, and beautiful as well.

The company is now taking these design strategies into the future, with a new-generation chair. The patient lying in bed, like a monarch on a throne, is the very essence of our image of a hospital room. But research shows that getting patients moving and exercising as soon as they are able reduces complications from blood clots and promotes good health. So Herman Miller designers have created a chair for use when the bed isn't needed. Like a twenty-first-century version of Alvar Aalto's Paimio chair, combined with a medical version of the Eames recliner, it is ergonomic, providing maximum comfort for the patient, but has features that allow easy access for caregivers. Sleek and modern in design, it is covered with antimicrobial, moisture-repellent, and easily cleaned yet aesthetically pleasing fabrics, and looks like it should be in a living room rather than a hospital room.

At Steelcase, new work-station modules are being developed for staff members, to increase their efficiency, minimize their stress, and reduce back injuries. They are also designed to increase the frequency and quality of staff-patient interactions. Joyce Bromberg, a vice president at Steelcase and one of the principle supporters of Steelcase's involvement in the Pebbles Project, now also a board member of ANFA, has developed a way to analyze nurses' work-flow patterns to document whether these innovations reduce unnecessary steps. Nurses are videotaped as they go about their tasks, and the films are analyzed according to a process called *video ethnography,* in which researchers trace the movements of healthcare workers through the hospital environment.

Video ethnography, though a new concept in healthcare design, is not new in the field of design in general. In 1926–27, at the height of the Bauhaus movement in Germany, the designer Grete Lihotzky collaborated with film director Paul Wolff to demonstrate the advantages of the modern, "rationalized" kitchen she had created. The black-and-white film shows a grim-faced older woman wearing a dowdy dress and apron, her hair pinned up in a bun, squandering her energy in an old-fashioned, inefficient kitchen: she runs back and forth between chopping block, wood stove, table, and sink. The scene then switches to a fashionable young woman wearing a flapper-style dress, her hair bobbed, happily cooking in her modern galley kitchen—a sleek affair with gleaming countertops, built-in cabinets, and smoothly gliding drawers. Sitting comfortably on a stool, all she has to do is turn her body in order to reach the utensils she needs. Then comes a schematic aerial view of the track each woman makes, superimposed on an architectural drawing of each kitchen. Clearly, the young woman accomplishes her task with less movement and effort.

This aerial view is similar to the perspective that Bromberg takes to calculate efficiencies of movement through video ethnography. Her analyses show that in standard centralized nursing stations, nurses zigzag here and there, often doubling back multiple times to accomplish a task. The units designed by Steelcase include furniture and modular countertops that have adjustable heights and varying widths, and can easily be arranged so as to optimize function. In patient rooms and waiting areas, furniture is likewise flexible and movable, providing comfortable seating for family and visitors. Trundle beds can be pulled out for family members who want to stay overnight. All this, together with the warm, soft earth tones and textures of the furniture, reduces the barren feel of the hospital environment and will go a long way toward reducing stress and isolation.

Professionals at the leading edge of healthcare design and architecture are joining with physicians, psychologists, nurses, and hospital administrators to incorporate such elements into the healthcare environment. Roger Ulrich and Craig Zimring have proposed a list of design changes that would improve patient safety by reducing infection, falls, and medical errors; mitigate stress; and promote healing. These include the use of single-occupancy rooms that could be adjusted to the medical needs of their occupants; improved air quality and ventilation; use of sound-absorbing ceiling tiles and flooring; better lighting and access to natural light; creation of pleasant, comfortable, and informative environments to reduce stress and provide patients, staff, and families with comfort zones, including gardens, nature views, and rooming-in spaces for families; making hospitals easier to navigate; and improving features such as nursing stations so as to help the staff do their jobs. Materials scientists are also developing new products which are easy to clean and make it difficult for germs to adhere to surfaces, yet are also acoustically absorbent.

Neuroscience research will lead to further innovation based on what we've learned about sensory perception: visual perception of depth, light, color, objects, scenes, and landmarks; auditory perception of sounds and silence; aroma recognition; navigation; and the effects of meditation and belief on healing. Designing hospital environments that support all of these brain functions will aid the body's own healing processes. By reducing the burden of stress and anxiety each patient carries, and by providing design elements to overcome deficits in perception and memory, these innovations promise to reduce medication dosages, surgical and medical complications, accidents, and error rates. Ultimately they will enhance a sense of well-being, speed healing, and prolong independence for the elderly.

An exciting frontier is developing at the interface between neuroscience and technology, in which knowledge of the way we perceive space, and of how we move around in it when we're healthy and when we're ill, is improving hospital design. Advances in this area are being applied to problems of way-finding and navigation in people whose memories are impaired. In a collaborative project involving the University of Pittsburgh, Carnegie Mellon University, the University of Michigan, and Stanford University, healthcare researchers and engineers are developing robotic nurses to help cognitively impaired patients navigate their environment. These "Nursebots" are walkers equipped with a laser-guided global positioning navigation system. A "smart" walker not only tells patients where they are in space and provides a topographic map of the location, but also learns their usual walking routines and guides them to their destination. The goal is not to replace nurses and caregivers, but to give individuals more independence in navigating their environment. Since independence enhances a sense of control, it also reduces stress.

In another initiative, a team of neuroscientists, computer scientists, and engineers at the University of California in San Diego (UCSD) are working together to develop portable EEG equipment to monitor the brain's electrical activity as a person navigates through real or virtual space. The idea of using mobile brain-imaging technology to understand way-finding in architectural spaces was the brainchild of Eduardo Macagno, the founding dean of biological sciences at UCSD. He already knew of the university's cutting-edge technologies in virtual reality and brain-wave analysis when he was invited to attend the first ANFA Woods Hole workshop in 2002—the same one at which Roger Ulrich discussed his work on healing views of nature. Macagno, a neuroscientist by training, had been assigned to the workshop's way-finding group. He raised the possibility of combining architects' expertise in designing virtual spaces with neuroscientists' ability to measure the brain's electrical activity in three dimensions. The goal would be to identify the brain's reactions to particular features of the built environment as a person navigated through a structure, even before it was built. This was an idea that had been percolating in his head ever since he'd learned of the StarCAVE technology being developed at Calit2 (the California Institute of Telecommunications and Information Technology).

Based on a design originally developed at the University of Illinois in Chicago, the StarCAVE is a virtual-reality system in which images are back-projected onto screens on the walls and floor of a multifaceted structure; the technology uses two projectors at each surface, angled and set exactly as far apart as a person's eyes. The participant wears polarizing glasses that filter out one image in the right eye and the other image in the left eye. The resulting effect is one of total immersion in a three-dimensional space. Because the participant uses both hand-held and head-mounted tracking devices (the latter device is attached to a small baseball cap), the scene changes in synchrony with the person's movements.

Such virtual-reality environments have been used for many purposes; the best-known is pilot training via flight simulators. The novel twist in the case of the Calit2 setup is the merging of sophisticated brain-imaging methods with the virtual-reality technique. It took several years for Macagno to get all the elements in place to begin to try out his idea. Above all, he needed the right mix of people with the right expertise. One such person was Scott Makeig, a computational neuroscientist who developed a way of using an EEG device to detect the source of brain activity in mobile subjects. Another was Eve Edelstein, a neuroscientist also trained in architecture.

Makeig is a multitalented scientist who can think across disciplines in the universal language of mathematics. Using equations, he can solve problems like the one that has plagued neurologists for more than half a century, since the EEG was first invented: how to pinpoint the source within the brain where the electrical activity detected on the surface of the skull originates. Makeig developed a way to resolve the mysterious moving squiggles of the EEG into three-dimensional images that reveal the origin of their electrical signals.

Edelstein's early research focused on how the brain perceives sound. She set up a neonatal hearing-test program for the State of California, advised NASA on how to monitor hearing loss in space, and helped the U.S. Navy identify genetic risk factors for noise-induced hearing loss. But she had always had an interest in architecture, thanks to her architect father, Hal Edelstein. As she was growing up, Edelstein says, "I used to think that tablecloths were made out of blueprints—the dining room table was so often covered with them." Eventually she decided to make her hobby her career. She became involved with ANFA's workshops, and obtained a degree in architecture at the New School in San Diego—the school where ANFA founder Alison Whitelaw taught.

Edelstein is now at Calit2, fitting participants with the EEG cap and observing them as they negotiate virtual space. She works with students and other scientists to figure out the anatomical coordinates that correspond to each of the 256 electrodes on the cap, so that the brain-wave signals can be correlated in real time to the images projected on the screens as the subject moves about the virtual world. As Edelstein demonstrates the bathing-cap-like headgear, a tangle of colored electrical wires dangling from it, she laments that she herself has not yet been a subject, though she would dearly love to be one. But in order to volunteer, she would have to cut short the mass of thick red curls that threaten to engulf her face. And unlike the graduate student who sports a Mohawk for the cause, that may be further than she is willing to go, despite her dedication to science.

The goal of the experiments is to see what parts of the brain respond to exactly what features of architectural space, and how they do so. Does a feature frighten, excite, or calm? What about brain regions involved in memory of place? Are there certain cues in the environment—landmarks, shadows, colors, volumes, scale, contrast—which attracts the participant's attention and which might help people navigate an unfamiliar environment? The hope is that the technology may eventually be able to show whether there is a particular electrical signature for feelings of anxiety when a person is lost, or a pattern that signifies comfort in a familiar environment. It might even help people with Alzheimer's find their way around, or reveal how certain physical environments might trigger a relapse in a person recovering from addiction.

Virtual-reality technologies are also currently being developed by the military to treat post-traumatic stress disorder (PTSD) in soldiers returning from war. Early results suggest that repeated immersion in a virtual space designed to resemble the scene of the trauma is capable of reversing symptoms by up to 80 percent in just ten weeks—a remarkable cure rate, if these numbers hold up in larger trials. This level of effectiveness is in line with pooled analyses from dozens of studies performed over the years on three hundred subjects treated this way for a variety of phobias and anxiety-related conditions, including PTSD. Thus, built space, whether real or virtual, could someday serve as a powerful adjunct in the treatment of mental disorders which are triggered or worsened by physical surroundings.

Edelstein is now a senior vice president of research and design at HMC, a company that is applying this new technology to healthcare design. Not only will such research help scientists to learn more about how the brain works when we navigate, but it will also help architects to design healthcare facilities that aid way-finding. Such information will be especially important in designing healthcare facilities for patients whose ability to form memories of place is impaired.

Other researchers are currently investigating ways to design hospitals with mental prostheses—modifications of physical space that can compensate for lost mental capacities. Patients suffering from Alzheimer's frequently have impaired depth perception. This causes them to perceive lines on the floor as steps or cliffs. When they alter their gait to negotiate the illusory obstacle, they sometimes fall and sustain life-threatening fractures, especially of the hip. By adjusting the texture of the floor in assisted-living residences, designers can reduce misperceptions and the incidence of falls.

Other design elements like those of Waveny's Main Street—indoor roaming spaces with views of the outside, abundant landmarks for way-finding, direct sightlines from bed to bathroom—enable residents to maintain their independence longer. Another chain of assisted-living facilities includes a variety of features to help residents cope with their physical environment: wide hallways with contrasting views at either end so residents can orient themselves, landmarks such as a large fireplace, a garden that is accessible to residents and also safe because it is surrounded by a high fence. An article published in *The Gerontologist* in 2003 showed that residents of such facilities do better on standard measures of depression, aggression, and social withdrawal than those occupying hospital rooms in typical nursing homes.

Other features make use of lighting and sound to create meditative spaces in waiting rooms or in quiet areas. There may be cascades of water, soft lighting, plants, furniture in earth tones, natural materials like hemp and bamboo on the floors and walls. That such features are calming seems obvious, but research proving the health benefits of stress reduction is providing a data-driven rationale for architects to include them in their plans.

Scientists are also learning how different wavelengths and intensities of light affect the sleep-wake cycle and in turn the stress response. Such knowledge is leading to new recommendations for lighting in intensive-care units, where activity continues round the clock. Technologies that measure heart-rate variability are allowing researchers to assess the effects of light wavelength and intensity, and other aspects of built spaces, on different components of the stress response. Other technologies are being developed that can measure immune molecules and stress-related chemicals in sweat. For example, a barely perceptible patch can be worn on the skin of the abdomen for twenty-four hours, providing a way to measure immune and stress responses without the need for drawing blood. Such technologies will help to identify spatial features that may be stressful, activating, or relaxing, and to determine their effects on immune responses, so that particular design elements can be incorporated, removed, or enhanced.

New knowledge about the sense of smell and aromatherapy is being incorporated into hospital design, in a field called *environmental aroma*. Research at the Monell Center in Philadelphia is addressing how such technologies could be incorporated into public spaces. Since certain aromas are known to evoke pleasant memories, subtle mixtures of such scents from nature could be combined with ventilation system technology to provide a pleasant experience for hospital patients. Combinations of scents can be designed not only to mask unpleasant odors, but to evoke positive emotions. The approach is already being used commercially in hotels and other buildings, to set a relaxing mood for visitors.

This may all sound like a brave new world where intuition in design is being superseded by technology and robots. But it needn't be that way. A happy balance can be established between intuitive design and technological advances, to improve health, mood, and cognition and to foster a sense of well-being in hospital patients and staff.

The nineteenth-century effort to eradicate infectious diseases by altering the design of hospitals has its parallel on a broader scale: that of entire cities. Throughout history, far-sighted scientists and planners have tried to control contagion by making changes in the physical makeup of cities.

One physician in England in the mid-eighteenth century did more than almost anyone else to improve the urban environment. His methods of discovery are still used today to identify and slow the spread of emerging infectious diseases on a global scale. His observations almost single-handedly brought about the changes in urban design that improved public health and created the modern cityscape.

11

HEALING CITIES, HEALING WORLD

John Snow was to urban public health what Semmelweis and Holmes were to hospital hygiene and infection control. Born to a working-class family in York, England, in 1813, Snow attended the Hunterian School of Medicine in London. He made notable contributions in two domains of medicine: the epidemiology of cholera and the development of the anesthetic chloroform. Perhaps his renown in the latter domain, garnered in part because he attended Queen Victoria in two births, protected him from complete ostracism by his colleagues, who strongly resisted his theories about the spread of cholera.

The story of Snow's battle to stop and prevent London's cholera epidemics is a drama worthy of Hollywood—a hero fighting big industry, political power, and entrenched dogma to protect the little guy. At the height of the Industrial Revolution, cities were vile places, with high infant and adult mortality, especially in poor and working-class neighborhoods. Nineteenth-century statistics reveal a substantial "urban penalty" when it came to lifespan. In 1880, for example, urban areas in the United States had 50 percent higher mortality than rural areas—an appalling rate, if you consider that only 6 percent of the population lived in cities, a much lower percentage than in England.

The main cause of this excess in urban mortality was infectious disease—not only cholera but also endemic tuberculosis, influenza, measles, and smallpox, among others. The larger the city, the higher the death rate. U.S. Census surveys show that in the middle and late nineteenth century, New Orleans had the highest average death rate, even between epidemics (fifty deaths per thousand), with New York, Philadelphia, Baltimore, and Boston close behind (as many as forty-five per thousand). Diseases flourished as a result of many factors: overcrowding; poor sanitation; dilapidated, badly designed, or nonexistent sewers; lack of potable water; and streets filled with rotting refuse. The influx of rural and foreign laborers added to the problem, since they brought new infectious diseases and were less resistant than long-time residents to endemic infections. The "rural advantage" did not mean that country folk were more aware of hygienic practices; it was simply a result of the fact that they lived farther apart.

By the 1920s, the situation had improved and the urban penalty had disappeared. This was due largely to improved sanitation and public health measures that were instituted in the mid-1800s, even before germ theory had been conceived or fully accepted. At first the going was slow. The notion that infectious disease could be transmitted from person to person or through contaminated water ran counter to the prevailing dogma that infection stemmed from a miasma emitted by decaying organic matter, from the poor moral character of the populace, or from the judgment of God. Local rumor even attributed one epidemic to the sewer company's unearthing of a mass grave where Plague victims had been buried in the 1600s. If these were the causes of urban epidemics, there did not seem to be any logical reason for improving sanitation, laying sewers, developing freshwater sources, or reducing crowding.

John Snow first experienced cholera during the 1831–32 epidemic in Newcastle. By 1849 he had come to believe that the disease spread through contaminated water. This was thirty years before Robert Koch formulated his principles for deducing the cause of bacterial illness—thirty years before he identified the *Vibrio cholerae* bacterium that causes cholera. Snow had noticed that the only symptoms cholera patients exhibited were gastrointestinal—in particular, "rice-water" diarrhea that caused death by dehydration. He reasoned that whatever was causing the disease had to have entered through the mouth. He thought it likely that the "poison" multiplied in the gastrointestinal tract; and although he was aware that Leeuwenhoek's "animalcules" could be observed through the microscope in contaminated drinking water and in the victims' stool, he did not make the connection between these organisms and the disease. Nonetheless, he proposed that ingesting water contaminated with fecal material was the cause and that avoiding drinking such water could prevent the disease. Like a sleuth, he set about to prove his hypothesis.

London in those days was engaged in a great many public-works projects to improve sanitation. The sanitary-reform movement in Victorian England held that overcrowding in cities, defective sanitation, and air and water pollution caused disease. Some far-sighted firms, such as the Lambeth water-supply company, had begun to move their sources upriver, away from sewage effluents. Snow realized that the construction of a new water supply by the Lambeth company could furnish the data he needed to prove his theory, since the Lambeth water source was far upriver, away from the polluted part of the Thames used by the other company that supplied the South London area, Southwark and Vauxhall. Comparing the mortality from cholera in households supplied by the two companies, he found that mortality was eight-and-a-half times lower in households supplied by Lambeth than in those supplied by Southwark and Vauxhall. This information alone would have been enough to generate resistance in some quarters, and Snow's findings continued to antagonize people. Then, on September 2, 1854, he was called in to help investigate a new outbreak of cholera, in the Broad Street–Golden Square area of London's SoHo district.

The public-hygiene measures being instituted to reduce epidemics were the focus of much political debate, and the Golden Square outbreak came at an awkward time for the government agency charged with preventing and containing epidemics. In 1848, Parliament had passed the Public Health Act and had convened a temporary General Board of Health to oversee expenditures for sanitary improvements and to respond to and advise the government during outbreaks of disease. This board, which included lay members as well as parliamentarians, wielded its power vigorously; its many investigations provoked the ire of local businessmen and medical professionals. When its term was up, Parliament dissolved it, and on August 12, 1854, created a much smaller and weaker Board of Health, headed by a single member of Parliament, Sir Benjamin Hall. Hall appointed a number of advisors to oversee sanitation and investigate epidemics. These included leaders in the medical and public-health community, as well as noted microscopists and chemists with the expertise to evaluate contamination of air and water.

Scarcely a month later, the Broad Street epidemic broke out. Several groups were directed to investigate, including the Board of Health and a committee of the Parish of St. James, Westminster. Because Snow had already been studying cholera, he was called in to advise the Parish of St. James and was made a member of its investigative committee.

Upon interviewing residents in the area, recording the location of cholera deaths, and taking into account data shared by other investigators, Snow determined that there was a cluster of cases around the neighborhood pump situated on Broad Street. Although it is said that he drew his conclusions after marking the cases as dots or small bars, one for each death, on a street map of the area, in fact he was not the first to use this technique.

While Snow did use the maps to demonstrate his theories visually, the way scientists now use PowerPoint presentations, it was Edmund Cooper, working for London's Metropolitan Commission of Sewers, who drew the first map of this sort to determine the pattern of spread in the Broad Street–Golden Square cholera epidemic. This is now a method that is standard in epidemiology and that yields important clues to the origin of outbreaks and the transmission of disease. Snow seems to have identified the Broad Street pump as the source of the cholera outbreak by using deductive reasoning. He noted that all the victims in the area had obtained drinking water from the Broad Street pump. Most lived close to the pump and used it as their main water source; others, who lived farther away, drank from it occasionally. Residents also reported that at the start of the outbreak, the pump's water had a foul smell and a soapy scum on its surface.

Snow was so convinced that water from this pump was the source of the outbreak that he met with the parish authorities on September 7. The following day they removed the handle of the pump, preventing people from drawing water there. According to Snow's account in the *Medical Times and Gazette* on September 23, 1854, in the two or three days after the pump handle was removed, the number of new cases "became very few." He was careful to qualify this statement by saying that the number of cases had already been dropping by the time the handle was removed, and that it was impossible to say whether the disabling of the pump had hastened the end of the epidemic. But his conviction that the pump was the source of the epidemic turned out to be correct. The end of the outbreak following the closing of the pump was the first solid evidence that cholera is spread through contaminated water and that preventing the use of contaminated water could stem the disease.

Several additional pieces of information would have significantly bolstered Snow's case, had he known about them.

These were discovered by others on the parish committee and by members of the Board of Health. The parish investigation had identified the *index case*—the first victim of the epidemic: an infant girl who lived at 40 Broad Street who had died from diarrhea on September 2. Her mother had washed her soiled diapers in the house sink. Investigators discovered that the house drains were inches away from the Broad Street pump, and that both systems were so deteriorated that sewage water from the drains seeped into the pump's drinking water. Another piece of information came from Edmund Cooper's map of the neighborhood's streets, pumps, and sewer drains: Snow had originally placed the Broad Street pump in the wrong location, not directly next to 40 Broad Street, as Cooper had done.

Yet Snow correctly interpreted the data, and his actions probably hastened the containment of the outbreak. In contrast, despite their more complete information, the Board of Health, possibly driven by the prevailing dogma in the medical establishment, soundly rejected Snow's theory concerning the waterborne nature of the disease. The board concluded that the cause was stagnant air, high barometric pressure, and the high temperature of the Thames water at night, and that the disease was spread through the air, not through drinking water. One piece of evidence that might have misled the board was supplied by the microscopist Arthur Hill Hassall, who examined the water of Southwark and Vauxhall and found it to be contaminated with the same cholera microbes that were present in victims' stool, while the water from the Broad Street pump was clean. This was probably due to the fact that by the time Hassall examined the Broad Street pump water, the point source of its contamination—the stool from the infant's dirty diapers—had long since washed away.

For some time afterward, public-health measures to contain

epidemics continued to include spreading lime on the streets, but did not advise minimizing contact with contaminated materials or infected people. Not until thirty years later, when germ theory was accepted and Koch had proved that cholera was caused by those bacteria the microscopists saw in the water, did the government institute public-health measures based on clean drinking water, well-built sewers, and lower population density.

John Snow received little credit from the medical community for his ground-breaking discoveries about cholera. His obituary in the *Lancet* in 1858 was brief and made no reference to them, although it did mention his work on chloroform. The reason for this neglect perhaps lies in a human failing of Snow's: he may have been so wedded to his theory of the waterborne nature of cholera that he discounted the possibility that other diseases could be spread through the air.

His confidence led him to testify before a parliamentary commission on behalf of the "offensive trades," whose production processes fouled the city air. Such businesses were involved in activities like boiling animal bones to produce soap, and slaughtering horses and livestock for their hides. In response to questioning from the committee, Snow repeatedly said he did not believe that these trades were in any way responsible for causing disease, and that the offensive odors they generated from rotting animal flesh posed no harm to humans. By defending the trades, he alienated the editor of the *Lancet*, a crusading medical journalist who felt that their practices should be more tightly regulated. As a result of all these factors, Snow's reputation within the medical profession suffered.

Despite the many advances in urban design since John Snow first observed the effect of cholera in London, the poor districts of the world's cities continue to have higher mortality rates than more privileged neighborhoods. Yet the greatest killer of the young in today's inner cities is not infectious disease but violent crime. And the illness that exacts the greatest toll is not cholera but asthma, whose incidence is rising. No one knows exactly why, but it could be related to increased exposure to dust mites and cockroach protein, compounded by parents' tendency to keep their children indoors as a protection against violence. Some people have proposed that a factor exacerbating asthma might be the stress attendant on living with the threat of violence and the hardships of poverty. Most likely, however, it is fueled by exposure to air pollutants. There is no question that the air in such environments is unhealthy.

Throughout history, people have associated cities with air pollution and poor health, and have attempted to correct or avoid these problems. Around 400 B.C.E., the Greek physician Hippocrates decried the foul air in cities and in 61 C.E., Seneca wrote: "As soon as I escaped the oppressive atmosphere of the city [Rome], and from that awful odor of reeking kitchens which, when in use, pour forth a ruinous mess of steam and soot, I perceived at once that my health improved." In 1170, the Hebrew physician Maimonides said: "The relation between city air and country air may be compared to the relation between grossly contaminated filthy air and its clear, lucid counterpart."

In the thirteenth century, English brewers and blacksmiths started to use bituminous coal harvested from outcrops along Britain's northeast coast. Later most people used it for heating and cooking. The famous fogs of London and other British cities were beginning even then, and became an annoyance to the nobility. In 1257 Queen Eleanor complained that Nottingham was too smoky and she moved to nearby Tutbury Castle, where the air was cleaner. By 1285, London had set up a commission to try to solve the problem. Edward I temporarily eased the situation by banning the use of coal, but that did not last long. In

1578 Elizabeth I once again banned the use of coal, but only when Parliament was in session.

Things deteriorated even more during the Industrial Revolution. In 1819 a Select Committee was established to look into the problem, and required that furnaces and engines be built to reduce the risk of pollution. In 1843 a second Select Committee was established with the same goals, but again nothing was done. In 1845 a third Select Committee concluded that there was no solution to the problem. In 1873 a series of dense, stifling fogs descended on London. These were in fact not fog, but thick smog that blanketed the city as a result of countless coal fires. The haze could be seen for miles around. Charles Dickens, in 1845, in the opening passage of *Bleak House*, described it thus: "smoke lowering down from chimney-pots, making a soft black drizzle, with flakes of soot in it as big as full-grown snow-flakes—gone into mourning one might imagine for the death of the sun."

Thousands of deaths were attributed to these fogs, the worst of which came in the mid-twentieth century: the acrid "Big Smoke" of December 1952, which blighted the city for five days and caused an estimated 4,000 deaths—a number that may actually have been three times higher.

The climatic conditions that foster smog are called *thermal inversions,* which occur when cool, heavy air is close to the ground and is prevented from rising by a layer of warmer air above it. The cold air is trapped, and the smog particles along with it. These conditions are of course not limited to London. Southern California, especially Los Angeles, is notorious for its smog. The first report of smoky air in Los Angeles was in 1542, from the Spanish explorer Juan Rodríguez Cabrillo, who noted when he sailed into Los Angeles Bay that the smoke from Native Americans' fires on the shore rose to a certain altitude and then spread laterally. It had apparently hit such an inversion. He named the harbor the "Bay of Smokes." Other smoggy cities include Mexico City, Buenos Aires, Beijing, Cairo, Seoul, Jakarta, and São Paulo.

Pollution in cities certainly has a negative impact on health. The World Health Organization estimates that polluted air is associated with 600,000 deaths worldwide every year. Ozone accumulations associated with air pollution can lead to more frequent asthma attacks. Studies in Southern California show that chronic exposure to these pollutants can damage airways in the lungs and is associated with increased incidence of lung cancer and deaths from heart and lung disease, even in nonsmokers. So when London's Board of Health linked bad air to the spread of disease, it was correct. Besides damage from smog, contagions such as tuberculosis are also spread through the air, and the crowded conditions in late nineteenth-century cities contributed to the prevalence of airborne as well as waterborne diseases. Many turn-of-the-century urban-renewal projects focusing on fresh air, sunlight, and decreased population density helped to reduce the spread of airborne illnesses. Of course, the advent of antibiotics helped even more.

Tuberculosis, thought to have been eradicated in the late twentieth century, is unfortunately making a comeback in the inner cities of America. The poor, the homeless, and the drug-addicted often discontinue tuberculosis therapy before completing a full course. This has led to the rise of antibiotic-resistant bacteria, which can spread in densely populated neighborhoods and during airplane travel.

With the recognition that urban conditions promoted infectious diseases, governments instituted measures to reduce air and water pollution, decrease population density, improve sanitation, and do away with areas of standing water, the breeding ground for mosquitoes and other vectors that carry disease. Gradually, these measures did improve urban health. Today, although the inner cities still struggle with health problems, wealthier neighborhoods now show a significant "urban advantage" in terms of health and lifespan.

This urban advantage is paralleled and amplified by an increasing rural and suburban penalty. In the twentieth century, millions of people fled the cities. Especially in America, they built suburbs whose design has generated its own health risks. Just as the shift toward sterility in hospitals created an array of health problems resulting from inattention to the emotions, changes in urban design did so as well. The isolation and long distances needed to travel to amenities, requiring automobile transportation, are a setup for illnesses such as depression and obesity and their attendant illnesses, such as heart disease, diabetes, and stroke. So as risk factors have increased in rural and suburban areas and decreased in cities, the latter have gained a distinct health advantage.

In 2007, New York City's Commissioner of Public Health released a report indicating that New York was now the healthiest place in the nation. People who were born in New York in 2004 are likely to live nine months longer than those born elsewhere, and life expectancy has increased faster there than anywhere else in the country: a whopping 6.2 years since 1990, compared to 2.5 years for the rest of the country. Who could have imagined that New York would be a healing place? The immediate association that comes to mind when one thinks of Manhattan is stress—from noise, crowds of people, swarms of cars, bright lights, and sensory overload of all sorts. Positive adjectives linked with New York might include exciting, stimulating, fast-paced, competitive—but not healing.

Yet Manhattan has a surprisingly low percentage of obese residents. A 2004 New York Health Department report shows a map of New York State, first published in 2004 in the *Journal of the American Medical Association,* in which each county or borough is color-coded, from white (lowest percentage of obesity) through gray (intermediate percentages) to black (highest percentage). In contrast to every other locality in the state, Manhattan is coded in white: only 10–14 percent of Manhattanites are obese. Prevalence rates of obesity in the rest of the state range from 15–18 percent on Long Island, to 20–24 percent in the other boroughs and in most of the rest of the state, to more than 25 percent in some counties upstate.

The Centers for Disease Control has likewise mapped the spread of obesity across the entire country. On the agency's website (CDC.gov), you will find a series of maps of the United States based on records that have been kept since the 1980s ("U.S. Obesity Trends, 1985–2007"). The evidence is dramatic and frightening. As the decades progress, there is a steady march of red across the map, the color indicating a high incidence of obesity: 25–29 percent. This red stain spreads from southeast to the north and from the Midwest out to the coasts. The map starts in 1986 with mostly cool blue, representing less than 10 percent obesity in most states, and by 1991 has gradually shifted to green (10–14 percent). By the mid-1990s, greens are turning to yellows and yellows to orange as the numbers shift to 20–24 percent in most states. By the 2000s, the oranges turn to red. On the last, the one for 2007, a couple of purple states crop up in the Southeast—purple representing an obesity rate of greater than 30 percent. One is left wondering where this trend is headed. Will purple take over the entire map?

What is omitted from this representation is that obesity not only seems to be spreading from southeast to north and from the central plains outward, but it also predominates in rural areas and in the suburbs. If one were to overlay a map of urban sprawl onto the map of obesity, it would be an almost perfect match. Urban sprawl is most prevalent in the Southeast and Midwest, where obesity is likewise most prevalent. Obesity is less common in the more compact urban areas; and the most compact cities, like New York, seem to be relatively immune.

There could be many reasons for the urban advantage, including proximity to wealth, with the associated spillover of better infrastructure, access to quality healthcare facilities, and a greater variety of foods and amenities. It could result from the closer social networks that exist in cities, or from physical factors that foster healthier lifestyles, such as increased exercise. It might be due to all of these factors.

Some researchers have proposed that thinner people who like to walk choose to live in New York City, and heavier people who prefer to drive choose to live in the suburbs. On the other hand, it could be, as most researchers propose, that the built environment in cities encourages walking, whereas the features of the suburbs discourage it. The very characteristics that make New York grate on your nerves—traffic congestion, lack of parking spaces, lack of cabs just when you need them—may be at the root of this health phenomenon, because place shapes behavior. No amount of telling people to leave their cars at home and walk will have an effect as powerful as these incentives not to drive. Since Manhattan is so compact and so filled with interesting sights, walking is far preferable to public transportation. And it is far less stressful, since you are in control. You know that you will get to your destination on time. You just need to wear a comfortable pair of shoes. Urban-design studies have shown that something as minor as the variety of details and finishes on buildings can encourage walking, and New York has these in abundance.

Safety is of course a concern when one is walking, but certain features can enhance safety—adequate lighting, shops, other people on the streets, and the physical condition of the neighborhood. The availability of sidewalks also encourages walking, and proximity to parks is a big factor in how much people use them.

New York has many parks—nearly all residents have one within walking distance of their home. With the 1980s drive to clean up these green spaces, rid them of trash and graffiti, and clear out drug dealers, the parks can now be used for socializing, sports, and dog walking, all of which are healthful activities.

Simply doing errands in New York involves exercise. And the legendary bustle of the New York way of life appears to contribute to health. New Yorkers walk faster than other people, and when they run their errands and hurry to work, they are doing so at the pace of a power-walker. Speed of walking has been shown to be an important factor in weight reduction and health; faster walkers show a greater health advantage. It seems that Manhattan is one enormous gym, with plenty of opportunities to work out in the course of one's daily routine.

Interesting landmarks encourage people to walk toward them. Disney theme parks call them *attractions;* urban planners call them *attractors.* These don't have to be as exciting as a fairytale castle. A study of St. Mark's Square in London showed that people tended to walk around the square from lamppost to lamppost, rather than cut across the square diagonally, which would have been the shorter distance. A study of a Montreal marketplace found, not surprisingly, that people walked toward pleasant and interesting things.

The type of study that defines the relationship between human behavior, layouts of cities, and forms of buildings is called *space syntax.* Such studies, which involve complex computer modeling, show that certain features of cities and of urban buildings are more conducive to making people walk. A feature called *integration,* a measure of how the local properties of a space relate to the surrounding city, is highly correlated with increased walking. The more interesting things to do and see in such spaces, the more people will walk, especially if they have many choices and more than one possible path to follow. Building-setbacks from the street are also important; older buildings, constructed before 1950, tend to be closer to the street and have storefronts opening onto the street, factors that encourage walking in cities like London and New York. Amenities like benches, water fountains, and bike racks also contribute to more walking.

Just as there are features of the urban landscape that encourage walking, there are features of the suburbs that discourage it and instead encourage driving. Long, winding streets ending in cul-de-sacs, lack of sidewalks, sameness of vistas, lack of activity and interesting sites, sprawl, long distances from residential areas to local shops and amenities—all characterize the suburban environment and discourage walking.

Besides correlating with obesity, the layout of suburbs and rural areas is associated with other health risks. The very factor that led to the rural advantage in the 1800s—lower population density—is now bringing other health problems. Isolation and lack of social support increase the risk of depression. As social support networks become denser, people become healthier. Professional healthcare is also less accessible in rural areas than in urban ones. Even when one takes socioeconomic factors into account, the rural poor fare worse than the urban poor.

While living in cities may confer a health advantage, the cities themselves are increasingly having a deleterious effect on the landscape and climate around them. This situation is introducing a whole new set of health problems on a regional and global scale. Cities are in fact contributing to the spread and emergence of a variety of diseases, because they disrupt the surrounding ecosystems. Urban sprawl, and the forest fragmentation that comes with it, are causing wildlife such as deer to forage for food closer and closer to human habitation. Such proximity brings greater exposure to contagions like Lyme disease, which is spread by ticks that live on deer. Characterized by a skin rash, arthritis, and neurological symptoms, Lyme disease was named after the town in Connecticut where the first North American case was recognized. It is now endemic in the suburban areas of the Northeast.

Deforestation and the draining of swamps is also removing important buffers which previously protected cities from severe weather. Part of the reason Central America sustained so much damage from Hurricane Mitch in 1998 is that deforestation led to mudslides. And the removal of wetlands around New Orleans, which were valuable as shock absorbers during storm surges, is thought to have contributed to the city's vulnerability to flooding during Hurricane Katrina.

Cities change weather patterns and weather-related health risks in other ways as well. The "heat island" effect causes cities to have considerably higher temperatures than the surrounding countryside. In some cities, such as Dallas, temperatures can be as much as ten degrees Fahrenheit higher than the surrounding countryside. Besides directly affecting the health of residents, especially those who cannot afford air-conditioning during extremes of heat, such conditions can also lead to inversions that trap pollutants. Airborne particles, nitrogen oxides, and sulfur oxides are harmful to the lungs. These conditions can predispose people to cardiovascular and respiratory diseases, which may be life-threatening for the elderly, the infirm, and the very young.

Cities also amplify weather patterns that can worsen pollution and contribute to global warming. Large cities can change the weather around them by creating plumes of warm air mixed with concentrations of pollutants. Increased precipitation and more frequent lightning were reported downwind of sixteen U.S. cities in 1995, changes which may have been due to this effect. Conversely, decreased precipitation has been reported in the wake of large cities in the United States and Israel. It is pos-

sible that these effects of cities on regional weather could cumu-
latively have a larger impact on global climate, especially if
urbanization continues. And by the middle of the twenty-first
century, 80 percent of the world's population is expected to be
living in metropolitan areas, particularly in Asia.

If the nineteenth century was the era of urban epidemics
and the early twentieth was the era when these were cleaned
up, then the twenty-first century will be the era of infectious diseases whose spread is increased by global warming and climate
change. It will be the responsibility of political leaders and health-
policy experts to correct the infrastructure and conditions that
foster such diseases related to global warming.

A 2007 report by the World Health Organization's Intergovernmental Panel on Climate Change focuses on the role of climate change in health. In a lecture at the National Institutes of
Health in the same year, the director-general of the WHO, Dr.
Margaret Chan, stated: "Climate defines the geographic distribution of infectious diseases, and weather determines their severity." Climate change, according to Chan, "is the defining
health issue of this century."

The WHO's 2007 report includes global maps which starkly
highlight this problem. A map in shades of orange through purple shows surface temperatures in oceans and continents, which
are projected to rise as much as seven degrees Celsius by the end
of the twenty-first century. Such rises in ocean temperature are
already contributing to the spread of infectious diseases, notably
cholera.

One researcher who has used maps on a global scale to prove
this point is Rita Colwell at the University of Maryland at College Park. Colwell is effectively the John Snow of the twenty-
first century. A quick, wiry woman with short gray hair and wire-
rimmed glasses, she pulls no punches. Her work linking the
spread of cholera to plankton in rivers and estuaries and to rising

ocean temperatures was the first to link climate change to the spread of infectious disease. Her findings were published in the *Proceedings of the National Academy of Sciences* in 2000, when global warming was not yet on the radar screen of most biological scientists or the general public. Her training in bacteriology, genetics, and oceanography positioned her perfectly to see the connections.

The methods she used were similar to the ones that John Snow and Edmund Cooper used to map the 1854 London cholera epidemic, but instead of doing house-to-house surveys, Colwell made use of data gathered by remote-sensing devices such as satellites, and thermal-mapping data collected by high-resolution thermal infrared aircraft. These could detect subtle changes in sea temperature, sea surface height, and chlorophyll concentration in oceans across the globe. The data could then be compared with one another and with regional infectious-disease statistics, with the aid of software programs collectively known as the Geographic Information System (GIS).

The region Colwell chose to study, Bangladesh and the Bay of Bengal, is one where cholera outbreaks occur regularly in spring and fall. Color-coded satellite maps of sea temperature throughout the year show a dramatic increase in red (indicating the warmest water temperatures) streaming across the bay in April and May, with yellow (the next-warmest temperatures) predominating in March and lingering through June. September and October are less dramatic, but still show warmer water temperatures compared to the winter months. Sea surface height has a similar ebb and flow across the seasons, as do chlorophyll concentrations.

Colwell and her colleagues at the International Centre for Diarrhoeal Disease Research in Bangladesh were able to map the cholera cases occurring in the region, and layer them on top of the environmental data. The patterns of variation in the numbers of cholera cases and the patterns in these ocean variables matched almost exactly. This was the first clear demonstration on a large scale that human infectious disease is influenced by climate patterns. The London Board of Health's observation in 1854 that water temperature contributed to cholera outbreaks was, it seems, not unfounded. The Thames is an estuary that is closely connected with changes in the sea—changes which could include water temperature and sea height, just as in the Bay of Bengal.

Colwell knew it was important to measure chlorophyll because of another discovery that she had made several years before. Cholera bacteria need plankton in order to grow. Plankton are single-celled plants that float in the oceans. There are two general kinds. *Phytoplankton* resemble plants, make chlorophyll, and derive their energy from the sun. *Zooplankton,* which are more like animals, use phytoplankton as their food. Cholera bacteria attach to a type of zooplankton called copepods, and as a result the sea is a reservoir where cholera bacteria live all year round.

Colwell also knew that it was important to measure changes in sea surface temperature, because, just like plants on land, the ocean's phytoplankton require warm temperatures, nutrients, and sunlight. When ocean temperatures rise in spring and summer, these plankton reproduce in sudden surges known as blooms. Several other environmental factors, including increased nutrients from agricultural runoff of nitrogen-rich soil and fertilizers, and changes in ocean salinity, can also spur their growth. And when phytoplankton bloom, so do the creatures they nourish—the zooplankton and their hitchhikers, the cholera bacteria.

Last, it was important to measure sea surface height because when the seas are high, ocean water flows back up rivers and estuaries, increasing the likelihood of human contact with the cholera bacteria. By mapping and layering all this data over an enormous surface of the globe, Colwell was able to show a link between global environmental changes and infectious disease on a scale never before attainable. These methods are now routinely used to map environmental factors—in particular, temperatures related to global warming—with the spread of many other infectious diseases. The results are alarming.

The disease burden from other infectious agents fluctuates seasonally as well, as a result of temperature-related variations in the growth of their reservoirs. Malaria, Dengue fever, Rift Valley fever, Ross River virus, and St. Louis encephalitis (all borne by mosquitoes) and Hantavirus and Plague (carried by rodents) vary with temperature and rainfall; they increase when both are high, since mosquitoes and rodents flourish in moisture. In addition to seasonal variations, these illnesses show cyclical variations related to larger weather cycles such as El Niño—an increase in Pacific Ocean water temperatures that occurs on the average every two to seven years. Several outbreaks of viral infections have been linked to the increased rainfall and flooding which result from El Niño. One, an outbreak of Hantavirus, occurred in May 1993 in the Four Corners area of New Mexico, Arizona, Colorado, and Utah.

The outbreak began when a young man and woman died within a week of each other of a rapidly progressive respiratory illness. The woman was twenty-one years old and living with her nineteen-year-old fiancé, a marathon runner, until then in perfect health. Two days after she died from a respiratory illness, he came to the local emergency room with a one-day history of flu-like symptoms: fever, malaise, myalgias, chills, and headache. His physical examination was normal, and he had no cough or difficulty breathing. He was sent home on antibiotics, an antiviral drug, and acetaminophen. He continued to worsen and returned to the emergency room two days later, now with vomiting and diarrhea. His physical exam was again normal, and he was sent home on the same therapy. He returned one day later coughing up copious amounts of yellow sputum tinged with blood, a symptom accompanied by shortness of breath and an extremely elevated white blood count. Shortly thereafter he developed acute respiratory failure and cardiac and respiratory arrest. Attempts to resuscitate him failed. On X-ray and postmortem examination, he was found to have massive pneumonia throughout both his lungs. He had essentially drowned in his own secretions.

By June 7, 1993, a total of twenty-four persons, from thirteen to sixty-four years old, had developed a similar disease in the same geographic area, some of them relatives of the initial two. Most had been in good health. Seventy-two percent were Native American.

As luck would have it, a mammalogist, Robert Parmenter, who had been working in the region in the spring and summer of 1993, provided the clue that revealed the epidemic's cause. He had noticed a dramatic increase in the deer-mouse population, which had exploded to ten times its normal number because of an unusual set of climate conditions attributed to El Niño: six years of drought had preceded unusually heavy rains and snows. This had led to an increase in pine nuts and grasshoppers, which caused an increase in the population of the deer mice that fed on them. The deer mice, in turn, increased the reservoir of Hantavirus.

Global warming is also beginning to contribute to the emergence of infectious diseases in areas that were previously unaffected. In much the same way that Colwell used remote-sensing devices and GIS in her research, other scientists have calculated rainfall by noting which plants are photosynthesizing and which are not. This gives an index of moisture or rainfall in a given area. Such analyses are showing that diseases like malaria are marching up mountain slopes in Africa, occurring at altitudes that were formerly too dry and too cool to sustain them. The mosquito that causes malaria is now found in areas where it had previously been unable to grow. With increased moisture, new breeding grounds are established in places that used to be arid. Higher temperatures speed the rate at which the mosquitoes reach adulthood, the frequency with which they feed on blood, and the frequency with which they are exposed to parasites. Higher temperatures also speed the growth of parasites inside the mosquito. The reason the greatest increase in malaria is occurring in the African highlands is that, at low temperatures, even small rises in temperature have great impact on malaria spread. A compounding factor is that in areas previously unaffected by malaria, people's immunity is low, making them more susceptible to infection.

Diseases fostered by climate warming are also spreading northward and spreading out in time. Outbreaks are occurring earlier in the spring and lasting later into the fall. And massive epidemics of infectious diseases—usually diarrheal disease, which can kill thousands—are occurring in the wake of major weather disasters like hurricanes. Some predict that such extreme weather conditions will occur with greater frequency and intensity as global warming continues. The approximately ten thousand people who perished as a result of Hurricane Mitch died not only from the immediate effects of the storm but also from the infectious diseases that flourished in its wake. People living in poverty and in underdeveloped countries are the ones who suffer most.

What to do about all this? First, we must recognize the existence of these problems at every level—local, regional, and global. At the local level, when designing neighborhoods, towns, and buildings, we must take into account those features of the built environment which affect health and health-related behaviors. At the global level, we must identify those features of the built environment that contribute to climate change, and work to minimize them. While instituting these changes, we must also gather data to evaluate their effects on health.

Walt Disney was far ahead of his time when he designed Epcot Center in Orlando. Epcot is an acronym that stands for Experimental Prototype Community of Tomorrow. Disney envisioned the park as a place where experiments in urban design and advances in technology could be tested and showcased. He also designed a utopian town named Celebration, which was built in central Florida after his death. Many people cringe at the thought of living in such a controlled environment, but those who live there love it.

Disney imagined that he would create a utopia in which neighborhoods were clean and orderly, in which the environment was controlled, and where people would be happy. He died of lung cancer before he was able to achieve this dream. But a version of it persisted and became part of the fabric of American culture. For better or for worse, his greatest legacy was the Disneyfication of America—of shopping malls, neighborhoods, even whole towns.

This is particularly evident in shopping spaces. In the 1950s, before Disneyland opened, shopping malls were rows of businesses lined up along the highway. No landmarks, nothing striking or different to attract a customer. They resembled a strip of stores along a street, but there was no attempt to induce an emotional response in the passer-by.

Now shopping malls go to the other extreme. Stand at the foot of the escalator in many department stores of an upscale chain headquartered in Dallas, and you can watch children hanging on to their mother's hand as they glide up, teenagers talking on their cell phones cocooned in a separate world, shoppers with weary eyes and deadened stares. But as soon as the escalator carries them into the butterfly cloud hanging from the skylit dome, they all look up and smile, their eyes following thousands of threads hung with white and silver feather-butterflies and coin-like mirrors dangling from the ceiling. During the day, the butterflies shimmer in the sunlight; by night, they are lit from below—an evocation of childhood fantasies, of snowflakes and Narnia, Christmas and the *Nutcracker*'s sugar plum fairies.

Who can resist taking the escalator up just one more flight, to get closer to those thousands of fluttering wings. The display is cleverly designed so that only a few of the butterflies hang all the way down to the store's first floor. They're just enough to make you curious. As you climb, more and more threads crowd together, and by the time you reach the top you're in a blizzard of white and silver and mirrors, their reflected light dancing on the escalator walls. Then, just beyond the shimmering veil, you see clothing racks and merchandise displays. There is no question that the space shapes people's behavior and lifts their spirits. The display is meant to draw you into the store and put you in the mood to buy. And it works.

This sort of theatrical display, which sets a mood by means of visual, auditory, odor, and collective-memory cues, is used over and over in retail marketing, so much so that we take it for granted. Appalling as it may seem, such examples show that it is possible to design urban places that buoy people's spirits, induce people to walk, and encourage socialization. If we could apply these principles to urban design instead of just to theme parks and shopping malls, perhaps we could offset some of the negative emotional and physical health effects of the suburbs, and even improve health in the poorest areas of cities.

More and more suburban towns are being built on such principles. There are central squares where people can congregate; front porches where people can socialize with their neighbors;

shorter blocks, with sidewalks to encourage walking; good lighting; easy access to amenities on foot; mixed-use areas, including offices, businesses, residences, and recreation centers; better
public-transportation systems, to encourage walking and discourage driving; and bike paths, tennis courts, parks, and golf
courses within easy access to the town center. Even the sheer cement walls of shopping malls are being "bumped out" so that
windows and entrances open onto the street, to encourage walking. These towns are reminiscent of the old towns and villages of
Europe. We may not be able to reach Utopia with these designs,
but at least we will exercise more while getting there. By designing towns to encourage walking, we can reduce our dependence
on fossil fuels, reduce the negative impact of cities on climate
and the environment, and at the same time improve our health.

One such place is Atlantic Station, a self-contained urban
center in downtown Atlanta, which is being redeveloped on a
so-called brownfield—an urban space that used to be a toxic
site, in this case an abandoned steel mill built in 1901. Like a
real-world updated version of Epcot, one that Disney might
have hoped for but never achieved, Atlantic Station is being
turned into an ideal urban center where people can live, work,
and play without using their cars.

It was the brainchild of Brian Leary, a Georgia Tech student
who first proposed the idea in his Master's thesis. Perhaps because he was just starting out and had no notion of how monumental a task it would be, or perhaps because the timing was
right for a daring new approach to sustainable urban design,
Leary was able to make his blueprint a reality. He persuaded real
estate developers and an insurance company to take over the
138-acre site and turn it into a mixed-use property. According
to press write-ups, the community contains houses, townhouses,
condos, and apartments for 10,000 residents, workplaces for
40,000 people, retail stores, restaurants, theaters, eleven acres of

parks and green spaces, bike trails, wide sidewalks, "share" cars, and trolleys linked to Atlanta's rapid-transit system.

Leary, who is now Atlantic Station's vice president for design and development, explained in a 2007 interview for Emory University's magazine *Public Health:* "We looked at great urban neighborhoods across the world and figured out why they worked. Cities like Savannah grew at a walking pace. Atlanta grew at 55 miles per hour. Now people are tired of gridlock. We've built a community the way it was defined 100 years ago. People can get out of their cars and live close to where they work, shop, and enjoy restaurants and movie theaters and reach it all on foot. They can walk to where they like to walk rather than drive to where they like to walk. Convenience is important, but it's also a healthier way of living—physically, mentally, and emotionally."

This vision fit perfectly with the CDC's recommendations for redesigning the built environment to reduce obesity. Researchers at the CDC, also based in Atlanta, realized that Atlantic Station provided a perfect real-life laboratory to test exactly how such changes in urban design affect the health of people who live there. In 2007 the CDC, in partnership with Emory University and Atlantic Station's developers, launched a project called SWAT (Studying Walkability and Travel). Its aim is to gather data from residents in the Atlantic Station neighborhood.

The plan calls for two hundred participants to be assessed prior to moving in, and then again one year later. They would wear activity- and travel-monitoring devices over a five-day period, and fill out questionnaires about their health, travel, and activities during these periods. The hope is that the information garnered will yield evidence about how the built environment affects activity and exercise, and will provide guidance for future developments.

Indeed, if the study is achieved, its findings will build on a tradition of gathering objective data in urban environments, established by an earlier landmark study of residents in an inner-city housing project in Chicago: the Robert Taylor Homes. Researchers found that residents who by chance had been assigned to apartment units located near plots of green performed better on attention tests and coped better with major life problems than those whose apartments, though identical to the others, were near barren areas. In their report, the researchers remarked how these findings attest to the power of nature, known throughout the ages by philosophers like Henry David Thoreau: that "the presence of a few trees and some grass outside a sixteen-story apartment building could have a measurable effect on its inhabitants' functioning."

All this gives hope that building urban spaces for sustainable living will not only be good for the environment, but will also be good for our health. Studies like these support the mantra of the Green movement—"Think global, act local"—in a very personal way. What could be more personal than our health? We can each do our part to improve our local environments, and in so doing find our own healing places.

There are many ways to find your healing space. Sometimes it takes coming through a period of stress and hardship—even illness, as it did for me—to help you find your place of peace and healing.

12

HEALING GARDENS AND MY PLACE OF PEACE

My father and I sat on the terrace outside the kitchen door, eating breakfast early on a spring morning. He had propped a book against his oversized coffee mug, an old white china cup with the word "Dad" inscribed on it. I didn't have to leave for school for at least an hour, and my mother and sister were still getting dressed. My father looked up at me from his book and smiled as I ate my cereal.

"Listen . . . listen to the sounds of peace," he said. I heard a dog barking, birds chirping, the pock-pock of a volley on the tennis courts across the street. These sounds did not seem unusual to me. I heard them all the time. Not until many years later, after my father died, did I understand what they meant to him. He'd spoken those words in the mid-1950s, when the war in Europe was only a decade behind him—still so fresh in his mind that he could appreciate such quiet moments and revel in a sense of peace.

His favorite psalm was the Twenty-Third. Sometimes, after dinner, he would pull a Bible off the shelf and sit at the table and read it to my sister and me. Every once in a while, he would look up at us with a smile that contained both wisdom and calm.

> The Lord is my shepherd: I shall not want.
> He maketh me to lie down in green pastures:
> He leadeth me beside the still waters.
> He restoreth my soul. . . .

Yea, though I walk through the valley of the shadow of death,
I will fear no evil.

My father had walked through the valley of the shadow of death during the war, somewhere in a concentration camp in a place called Transnistria. I found that out after he died. He had never talked about it. I hadn't thought of my father as a religious man, and he wasn't—not in the organized-religion sense of the word. He never went to synagogue, never followed any of the Jewish rituals. But he was deeply spiritual, as I came to understand much later.

At the end of his life, he suffered a long and debilitating illness, akin to a combination of Alzheimer's and Parkinson's. It was a dreadful thing to watch: the slow inexorable decline in a man whose whole being had been centered on creative endeavors—conducting medical research on the peaceful uses of radiation, lecturing around the world, writing and editing.

A few days before his death, I stood in my kitchen with my daughter at my elbow, stirring a bubbling pot of kumquat jam on the stove. I had just returned from California with a bag of those fruits, so I'd decided to make the jam. The kitchen air was filled with its fragrance. It reminded me of my grandmother's kitchen, and me standing next to her, as my daughter stood now, eagerly waiting for the first sweet taste. We would drip the jam into a glass of cold water, to be sure it fell in tight globules to the bottom of the glass. That meant it was ready to pour into the waiting jars. Then the phone rang. It was my father's doctor in Montreal, telling me I'd better get there quickly. There wasn't much time. I threw a few things into a suitcase. As I headed out the door, I hesitated and went back into the kitchen for a jar of the jam. My father had always loved it.

When I got to Montreal and my father's hospital room, he was lying in bed, his breath rattling that deep, slow rhythmic pattern of death. He seemed asleep, or unconscious. I leaned over and whispered in his ear. He made no response, and his breathing continued uninterrupted. I stroked his forehead. It was sweaty. There was still no response. Finally I remembered the jam in my handbag. I pulled it out and reached for a spoon that lay on the night table beside his bed. As I opened up the jar, its sweet fragrance escaped and for a brief second masked the sour smell of his labored breath. I dipped the spoon into the jar and held a drop to his dry and pasty tongue. At first nothing happened, but then a smile slowly spread across his face. It was his last smile. He slipped away a few days later.

The terrace where my father and I had sat that summer day so long ago overlooked our garden—my mother's sanctuary. It was filled with flowers in the spring, summer, and fall, different plants coming into bloom in each season. Tulips, daffodils, tiny white snowdrops, and crocuses gave way to white trilliums and blue vinca. Then came the white and blue forget-me-nots (my grandmother's favorite flowers). The peonies, some deep pink, others white or red, were always filled with ants that tickled my nose when I tried to inhale the flowers' sweet scent. The irises in shades of iridescent purple also smelled sweet. They looked so stately with their furry yellow centers and knife-edged leaves, and towered over the purple pansies with their smiling yellow faces. I never much liked the orange tiger lilies—they were so scraggly—but my mother loved them, as she loved all the other plants. There were two kinds of velvety clematis that wound around each other as they climbed the fence post—one deep violet, the other a lighter shade. There were roses of many colors and sizes, spikes of light-blue monk's hood, pink and mauve phlox, and balls of white spirea hanging on their bushes like cotton wool. In early spring the odor of lilacs filled the air, and on summer nights the scent of mock orange blossoms and sweet white and purple alyssum drifted toward the house.

In the center of it all stood two cherry trees and an apple tree. In May and June I would lie in the grass beneath the cherry trees and gaze up at the clouds of white blossoms, watching them flutter to earth like snowflakes, sometimes catching them on my tongue. At the end of the summer, we climbed tall ladders to pick the yellow-tinged sour cherries hanging heavy from the branches. My mother fought a constant battle with the squirrels and birds to save the fruit, so she could cook it into pirishkas, a cherry-filled pastry she had learned to bake from her mother in Romania. My sister and I used to stand beside my mother in the kitchen, helping her cut the dough with a glass to make the circular forms that we filled with cherries, carefully pinching the edges together to shape the little pockets. We waited impatiently until they were baked, so we could eat them while they were still hot, and dripping with tart-sweet cherry juice.

In winter the garden lay dormant, covered with a deep layer of snow until late April, when bits of green started to poke through the dead leaves and branches. That's when my mother would spend hours in the garden, pulling weeds, trimming away dead brush, turning the muddy earth to make way for her beloved plants that soon would push forth from the soil. At the end of the day she would come back into the house with muddy boots and dirt-streaked face, looking tired but happy. In the summer she rejoiced when it rained, because her plants were being watered and nourished.

Gardens are peaceful places, little bits of re-created nature inside cities, or sweeping formal places carved out of wilder spots. Gardens have given people a place of respite since the beginnings of recorded history, and in legend, poetry, and song: the Garden of Eden, the hanging gardens of Babylon, the gardens along the ancient Silk Road of Persia, India, China, and Japan.

You can find gardens in the most surprising spots. In Washington, D.C., there is Dumbarton Oaks, where the treaty that launched the United Nations was signed. For more than a month in the summer and fall of 1944, representatives from the United States, the Soviet Union, the United Kingdom, and the Republic of China met at the mansion to hammer out the agreement. It was a fitting meeting place for the delegates, all from countries still at war who longed for peace.

The terraced Italianate garden was created in the 1920s. Depending on the season, you can wander through its winding paths past groves of forsythia, azaleas, and roses, or past colonnades of flowering plum trees and hills of ornamental cherry, crab apple, or dogwood; or you can sit on wooden benches under canopies dripping with purple wisteria, immersed in their sweet scent. When you are deep in the garden, you have no idea that you are just blocks from the center of Washington and the crowded streets of Georgetown.

In downtown Los Angeles you can find an even smaller space, a terraced Japanese garden that is tucked in a corner behind a hotel. It is three stories above the street, hemmed in on one side by the towering Caltrans building and on the other by the hotel. As you wander into the garden from the hotel's Japanese restaurant, you might think you are on a terraced slope. A Japanese maple and an ornate topiary guard the entrance to the garden. Straight ahead is a waterfall; nearby, a flight of stone steps leads to the top of what looks like a small hill. In fact, the "hill" and the waterfall cleverly disguise a step-like roof that forms the ceiling of the banquet hall below. This elaborately landscaped roof garden features a winding path that leads over and between many water features: a quiet little pond with sloping pebbled beach; the dramatic waterfall that splashes down an eight-foot wall of rock into another pond; a winding brook with stepping-stones and a little wooden bridge. Sitting at a bistro table in the shade of the trees at the back corner of the garden, you can hear the traffic sounds of honking cars and sirens mixed in with the gurgling of the little brook that courses through the space. Papyrus, cattails, tall grasses, and ferns edge the brook, along with pink and white impatiens and azaleas. You can smell mud and greenery, mixed with the smells of frying fish and beef from the restaurants in Little Tokyo. If you focus on the garden sounds and sights and smells, you can escape, if only for a moment, from the heat and rush of city life. Even seen from a window in the hotel high above, the garden provides your eyes with a respite from the glare and heat reflecting off the asphalt roofs and pavement down below. Indeed, this "green roof" cools and protects the building beneath it from the unrelenting sun.

Just northeast of downtown Los Angeles, in San Marino, is a Chinese garden, part of the Huntington Library complex founded in 1919 by railroad magnate and real estate developer Henry Edwards Huntington. It features many types of gardens from around the world, including a Shakespeare garden and a Baroque-style grande allée, complete with marble statues and fountain. The newest addition to the site, Liu Fang Yuan, or Garden of Flowing Fragrance, was built according to Chinese tradition. The indigenous trees—California oaks, tall spreading giants with tiny holly-like leaves—form a stately grove at the back of the landscaped pond. The water itself is located in a spot where water naturally accumulates after a heavy rain, in front of the grove of trees. Behind it all, the San Gabriel Mountains can be seen hugging the garden in the distance. Indeed, the layout of the garden follows the ancient tradition of Feng Shui, with protective mountains and forest at its back, and flowing water at its front. This arrangement, according to these principles, is best suited to keeping the Chi, or life force, flowing and harmonious. The garden is true to its name: fragrance, water, and life force flow throughout the space.

The formal section of the garden follows Chinese principles of harmony, and forms a striking contrast to the natural, untouched elements at its back. A series of walkways ring the pond, looping into small peninsulas and islands, each with their tiny slate-roofed pagodas, or larger, ornately carved wooden pavilions. The buildings provide shade and quiet spots to sit, think, meditate, or talk with friends. But they also provide many different views of the gardens, and of the mountains in the distance, framed through their latticed windows and walkways, arches, and wooden pillars. In the more open pagodas, you can feel the breezes and hear the rustle of the leaves in the surrounding trees. Or you can hear the bubbling source that feeds the shallow pool, and smell the jasmine and the pine.

The pond is edged with rocks from Lake Tai in China, rocks that are meant to evoke their mountains of origin and that symbolize the eternal—in contrast to the water, which symbolizes the ever-changing. The trees and plants around the edge also have their symbols: bamboo for flexibility and strength; pine for endurance, because it stays green all year long; plum for perseverance and courage, because it flowers even in harsh weather in the spring. As you lean over the railing of the arched stone bridges, you can watch the large golden, white, and orange-splotched Koi fish swimming lazily about.

A security guard, speaking fluent English with a thick Chinese accent, says that according to Chinese tradition, if you live in harmony with your surroundings, you're like a fish in water. Hence the name of one of the granite walkways over the pond: "Bridge of the Joy of Fish." He hesitates, then turns back to tell me more. Born in 1948, he was graduating from high school when Mao Tse-Tung started the Cultural Revolution. He and his comrades were sent to the countryside, where he spent five years laboring on a farm. His family suffered terrible hardships. In 1976 he escaped to Hong Kong, and then to the United States. He became an aerospace engineer, but frequent bouts of depression curtailed his career. He took up painting, but that endeavor, too, was cut short by flashbacks and depression. In the garden, he was healing—slowly coming back to life. His days were spent walking the calming paths around the pond, checking the grounds and helping visitors.

Still farther north from downtown Los Angeles, high on a hilltop overlooking the city, are the Getty Center gardens designed by architect Robert Irwin. A waterfall cascades from the walls of the museum, over boulders, down to a circular pool. The stream is criss-crossed by a walkway, a sharp zigzagging gash in the earth lined with rusting iron rails that contrast with the cool, quiet brook it traverses. The path takes you back and forth, from the shade of the trees to the baking sun, closer to then farther from the water's sounds and smells, so that you are keenly aware of your changing relation to each element around.

But gardens needn't be grand to be peaceful and inviting. They can be as tiny as a city lot containing only one or two trees. In downtown Chicago, just steps off North Michigan Avenue near the lake, you can stand in the courtyard of the Fourth Presbyterian Church, and the noise of all the traffic seems to disappear. Through the church's five stone arches, you can see the cars and people going by. But turn your back, and you're in another world. The lawn in the center of the space is just large enough to hold two tall spreading silver maples. The walkway around the perimeter is lined with low boxwood hedges and a few scattered flowers. In the middle of the space is a large stone fountain resembling the ones you can see along the Camino Frances on the way to Santiago de Compostela. A plaque on it says that it was donated by the architect of the church, Ralph Adams Cram, who also designed the Cathedral of St. John the Divine in New York. Water trickles from four spouts into an octagonal pool in a soothing understatement, its sound yielding to the birds that splash in it and accompany it with their songs.

Three weeks after my father died, I went to the Bishop's Gar-

den of the National Cathedral in Washington, D.C. It was a perfect evening on one of the first warm days in March. The cathedral and the garden are at the highest spot in the city. From
here, when the trees are not yet fully covered with leaves, you
can see the lights of the city twinkling through them far below. I
had come here, shaking with emotion, crying with uncontrollable heaves, in a way that I had not been able to since my father's
death. Earlier that evening I had attended a ceremony for the six
million Jews killed in the Holocaust—an annual event at which
my daughter, then ten years old, sang in the choir. This year's
event was different from those of prior years. It was held in a
synagogue and was modeled on a Jewish funeral, chants and
prayers and all. When, from my seat at the back of the darkened
hall, I heard the children's voices lifting sweetly up, my sobs began and didn't stop. I had to escape to someplace where I could
be alone.

As I stood and watched the city lights below the cathedral
garden, a warm wind came up and tossed the blossoms from the
weeping cherry that guards the stone moon-gate at the entrance
to the garden. The petals fell on me and swirled and eddied in
the curb, like the snow that had fallen in Montreal just three
weeks before, when we buried my father in the cemetery halfway
up the slopes of Mount Royal. Whether it was the similarity of
place, I do not know, but at that moment I felt his presence as
strongly as if he were alive, and with me under the cherry tree of
my youth. It reminded me of the times he had gently stroked my
forehead when I was ill, and I finally felt a sense of calm.

Six years later, my mother lay dying in the Royal Victoria
Hospital in Montreal. Next to her bed was a tall window that
Florence Nightingale would have approved of. It faced the
mountain and its dense woods, not the city side of the hospital,
and the ground sloped steeply upward. The snow was deep beneath the trees, and their branches, heavy with snow and ice,

sparkled in the sun. My mother mostly slept, but whenever she opened her eyes and her gaze fell upon those trees, she seemed at peace.

Three months after my mother died, I sat alone at the doorway of a tiny stone chapel on a hill overlooking the village of Lentas, on the southern coast of Crete. The lintel was so low that I had to stoop to enter the dark recesses of the chapel. But it was cool inside, and sitting there provided respite from the baking sun. The chapel smelled of musty stone and earth, and of wax from the many candles the villagers had lit next to the icons that filled the place. Sitting on the stoop, I squinted into the blinding sunlight. The opening framed a sweeping view of the land and sea and village, which hugged the hillside along a cove shaped by a hill that jutted out into the Mediterranean. It was the bluest sea imaginable, and looked even bluer in contrast to the white stucco houses of the village, framed by their red tile roofs and riots of fuchsia bougainvillea.

I had come here with my new neighbors, a Greek family, who had invited me to stay in their cottage in the village. Exhausted during the last months of my mother's illness, I had developed arthritis, with stiffness, pain, and swellings in my knees and wrists and shoulders. I had undergone all sorts of tests—biopsies, needle aspirations, and X-rays—to identify the cause. I was treated with medications but the symptoms persisted. I had planned to go back into hospital to try a new treatment, but delayed in order to come to Crete.

The little stone chapel where I sat was built on top of the ruins of a much larger Byzantine church, and it in turn atop an ancient temple to Asclepius, the Greek god of healing. Here, more than two thousand years ago, the sick would come to be healed with sleep, dreams, healthy diet, fresh water, music, exercise, and support from friends. They would climb the sloping ramps to the temple, just as I had climbed the pebbly paths, at first hesitantly, then with increasing confidence. From my perch I could sit for hours in quiet contemplation, looking at the view and watching the goats as they scrambled up the rocky slopes. I could listen to the silence, punctuated only by the occasional distant baaing of sheep, the twittering of birds, and the scritch-scratch of the gardener's rake as he tended the hallowed soil. For me, these were the sounds of peace.

We are all intimately connected to the place around us on a mi-cro and a macro scale. Our sense of place can come from some-thing as small as a drop of morning dew on a blade of grass, the smell of wet earth after a rain, or the sound of a sparrow skitter-ing across the pavement. It can come from the feel of gravel be-neath our feet or the warm sun on a bare arm. It can come from something as large as the image of the earth suspended in the black and silent vacuum of outer space. Our sense of place is cre-ated through what we see and feel and smell and hear—through all our senses. It is created and re-created in memory each time we experience and reexperience the place. Emotions, both good and bad, become attached to a place, which can then evoke myr-iad layers of feeling when we come back to it: the sense of calm that we call home; the thrill and anxiety that we associate with something new; the dread of reexperiencing trauma that once happened there; the longing for a love that we experienced there many years ago. A place can trigger unhappy memories or bad habits without our realizing it, and cause us to spiral down into drug addiction or despair. In turn, some places, which we have learned to associate with safety, can rescue us in times of need. Each of these emotions triggers cascades of nerve chemicals and hormones, which are released through the outflow pathways of the brain. These in turn change immune cells' ability to fight disease or heal, and all affect our health.

The people in a place also change its effects on health. Too many, and we may be crowded out and infectious disease may flourish; too few, and we may become isolated and depressed. Just enough and we have a secure network of social ties to help us through times of illness and of want. Illness, too, shapes our sense of place; it can color our emotions and blur our memories.

We are all part of our world, and what we do in the spaces around us not only shapes them but shapes our selves. We can create places that devour and destroy the environment and that in turn destroy us. Or we can do the opposite—create places that help us to live in harmony with the environment and sustain our health.

Architects through the ages have tried to do the latter: the ancient Greeks, who prized the "golden mean"; Christopher Wren, whose St. Paul's Cathedral captured sound; Frank Lloyd Wright and the Modernists, who created the light and airy buildings of the early twentieth century; Louis Kahn, who built the Salk Institute in alignment with La Jolla's ocean cliffs. An awareness of how place affects mood and behavior, and in turn our health, is helping today's architects design places that work with our bodies to maintain health and promote healing, rather than work against us to worsen stress and disease.

These principles are being applied to hospital design, which is merging elements that sustain both body and mind. These allow for reduction of noise while still keeping surfaces clean. They include spaces that permit isolation of patients to protect against infection, while providing room for family and friends. They offer soothing views of nature and just the right amount of light and color to create moods that can help heal. They take into account memory and perceptual failings of the patients and include elements that help them maintain independence. Unpleasant odors that carry with them the association of hospitals and disease are being replaced with pleasant scents. Technological innovations and carefully situated landmarks are easing navigation through the maze of hospital corridors, especially for the elderly and for those whose memories have failed. The need for exercise and physical activity is also being addressed, with innovations changing the very concept of the hospital bed.

Beyond the hospital, at a more global level, the knowledge that places can encourage walking and healthy exercise, or can discourage it and lead to obesity, has spurred a movement to design towns and cities so as to encourage exercise and social interactions. Just as the sanitation movement of Victorian times finally stopped epidemics of infectious disease, so should urban design incorporate features that encourage exercise and healthy living and control the modern epidemic of obesity. The new movement of sustainability, green architecture, and urban planning is helping to do just that.

As Alison Whitelaw drove me back to La Jolla after an ANFA meeting, past the Salk Institute and the Pacific Ocean, stars twinkling in the deepening evening sky, she confided to me what had really caught her imagination when she first heard of the potential for bringing neuroscientists and architects together. ANFA, she said, just seemed like the logical next step. We have all sorts of criteria for green buildings, but we're neglecting the effect on humans. We need the research to prove that such architectural elements are beneficial to people.

Neuroscientist Eduardo Macagno makes the same point about evidence-based design. What evidence do we need, and how do we get it? If we can observe brain function as people are experiencing the space, if we can find an integrated way to monitor all their brain and physiological responses, we might achieve an understanding of what works and what doesn't, and why. We can figure out how to promote learning, better health outcomes, better moods, or whatever the space is designed for. And we could design places to support people with deficits in memory or mental function.

One of the architects sitting in the front row when Eve Edelstein received the Best Sustainable Practices Award from the City Center Development Corporation of San Diego was Alison Whitelaw. Edelstein had received the award for "integrating sustainable ranking systems with human performance measures in an effort to make the human element visible and quantifiable as part of the effort to create truly high performance design." As Edelstein put it, "Effects on human performance matter as much as building performance, when it comes to green design."

This was effectively the question John Eberhard had asked me long ago in Washington, when we first met: "How can we measure people's responses to built space to improve their productivity and creativity, when what they are producing is a creative product that cannot be weighed and measured in numbers of widgets?" We have come a long way toward answering that question, but the going is slow and much more remains to be done.

The new frontier in architecture and urban design must take into account the needs of our emotions and the strengths and limitations of our brain's ability to synthesize the signals we receive through each of our senses. It must do this at every level, from small to large, from our immediate surroundings to a global scale. Research must ask *how* the brain responds to built space, and *whether* specific aspects of design affect specific aspects of health. And more research must be done on whether virtual or actual space, alone or as an adjunct to conventional drug therapies, can be used as a treatment for illnesses in which the environment triggers the symptoms.

This is the next step in shaping our environment beyond the basic bodily needs that were the focus of previous centuries. It goes beyond cleaning up hospitals and cities to rid them of infectious and toxic illnesses. It embraces a new notion of health that goes beyond the mere absence of disease and incorporates sustenance of the emotions as an essential part.

When I asked Ann Berger, the head of Pain and Palliative Care at the NIH Clinical Center, for her definition of healing, she said: "In palliative care, healing is thought of as a sense of wholeness. It is not being cured necessarily, but feeling whole. There is a difference between curing and healing, and what we do in palliative care is help people heal, no matter how sick they are."

The World Health Organization defines health as "a state of complete physical, mental, and social well-being and not merely the absence of disease or infirmity." The built environment affects all these aspects of health. Many organizations across many disciplines, including the health sciences, the healthcare professions, architecture, design, and urban planning, are working together to develop research programs that address this definition of health. In 2002, the Centers for Disease Control in Atlanta gathered representatives from these various groups to address several problems: how to study the effects of the built environment on health, how to determine the aspects of health that are influenced by the built environment, and how to address the needs of the system at all levels. In the same year, the National Academy of Sciences held a conference entitled "Green and Healthy Buildings for the Healthcare Industry." In 2005, the National Academies published a report of a workshop entitled "Implementing Health-Protective Features and Practices in Buildings," and many of its leaders from federal agencies, including NASA and the EPA, continue to work together as part of the Federal Interagency Committee on Indoor Air Quality. Many other organizations are now expanding these horizons to examine all aspects of the built environment on health: the CDC's studies of walkability and obesity are a prime example. The National Building Museum in Washington, D.C., has also taken up the charge, with an exhibition called "Green Community" that addresses many of these issues, including health.

Much research has come out of these plans and others like them, and more is yet to come. We are now at a threshold where we can apply new micro and portable technologies to measure brain, emotional, and immune responses to built space. Such measures will help to determine how the environment affects health. This information will in turn help us to identify ways to design space that can sustain health.

Organizations, large and small, well established or still in their infancy, are joining the challenge. Organizations like the Center for Health Design, and their Pebbles Project; the National Academy of Sciences, with their Healthy Buildings Project; the Academy of Neuroscience for Architecture, which focuses on the neuroscience of place; the Robert Wood Johnson Foundation; and the Agency for Healthcare Research and Quality are just some of the groups that are funding and investigating different aspects of this problem.

We can each, as individuals, do our part. Rather than rushing through our busy days without paying much attention to the spaces around us, we need to carve out a few moments here and there to allow ourselves to be aware of our place in the world and its place inside us. We need to allow ourselves the time to see the sun glinting off the surface of the leaves, to listen to the sounds of silence and of nature. We need to stop and inhale the smell of ocean salt or the fragrance of honeysuckle on a summer's night. We need to feel the gentle touch of a spring breeze. We can do all this whether we are healthy or ill. We need to let these sensations penetrate us, and take the time for the memories they trigger, both good and bad, to percolate to the surface of our thoughts. We need to let those memories take hold of our emotions and allow ourselves the time for reverie. Perhaps it was doing all of this that allowed those patients with views of nature to heal faster than those whose views were of a brick wall. It was only when I finally let go, and let the sun and sea and memories and emotions wash over me, above that tiny village in Crete, that I truly began to heal.

In this way, we can create for ourselves a place of healing—a tiny island—wherever we find ourselves in this world, at any moment in the interstices of our busy lives. It is really in ourselves, in our emotions and in our memories, that we can each find our healing space. For the most powerful of healing places is in the brain and in the mind.

BIBLIOGRAPHY

ACKNOWLEDGMENTS

INDEX

BIBLIOGRAPHY

1. HEALING PLACES

Campbell, M. (2005). "What tuberculosis did for modernism: The influence of a curative environment on modernist design and architecture." *Medical History*, 49 (4): 463–488.

Eberhard, J. P. (2008). *Brain Landscape: The Coexistence of Neuroscience and Architecture*. New York: Oxford University Press.

Gutheim, F. (1960). *Alvar Aalto*. New York: Braziller.

Hobday, R. (2006). *The Light Revolution*. Forres, Scotland: Findhorn Press.

Jardine, L. (2002). *On a Grander Scale: The Outstanding Life of Sir Christopher Wren*. New York: HarperCollins.

Kohn, L., J. M. Corrigan, and M. S. Donaldson. (2000). *To Err Is Human: Building a Safer Health System*. Washington, D.C.: Institute of Medicine, National Academy of Sciences, National Academies Press.

McCoy, E. (1960). *Richard Neutra*. New York: Braziller.

Molnar, Z. (2004). "Thomas Willis (1621–1675), the founder of clinical neuroscience." *Nature Reviews Neuroscience*, 5 (4): 329–335.

Ulrich, R. S. (1984). "View through a window may influence recovery from surgery." *Science*, 224 (4647): 420–421.

2. SEEING AND HEALING

Vision and Visual System

Hubel, D. H., and T. N. Wiesel (1962). "Receptive fields, binocular interaction and functional architecture in the cat's visual cortex." *Journal of Physiology*, 160: 106–154.

Logothetis, N. K. (1999). "Vision: A window on consciousness." *Scientific American*, 281 (5): 69–75.

Parker, A. J. (2007). "Binocular depth perception and the cerebral cortex." *Nature Reviews Neuroscience*, 8 (5): 379–391.

Shatz, C. J., S. Lindstrom, and T. N. Wiesel (1977). "The distribution of afferents representing the right and left eyes in the cat's visual cortex." *Brain Research*, 131 (1): 103–116.

Color Vision, Color Blindness, and Effects on Mood

Babin, B., and T. Suter (2003). "Color and shopping intentions: The intervening effect of price fairness and perceived affect." *Journal of Business Research*, 56: 541–551.

Field, M., and T. Duka (2002). "Cues paired with a low dose of alcohol acquire conditioned incentive properties in social drinkers." *Psychopharmacology* (Berlin), 159 (3): 325–334.

Hunt, D. M., K. S. Dulai, J. K. Bowmaker, and J. D. Mollon (1995). "The chemistry of John Dalton's color blindness." *Science*, 267 (5200): 984–988.

Schafer, A., and K. W. Kratky (2006). "The effect of colored illumination on heart rate variability." *Forschende Komplementarmedizin*, 13 (3): 167–173.

Sharpe, L. T., A. Stockman, H. Jagle, and J. Nathans (2001). "Opsin genes, cone photopigments, color vision, and color blindness." In L. T. Sharpe and K. R. Gegenfurter, eds., *Color Vision: From Genes to Perception*. Cambridge: Cambridge University Press.

Sherman, H. (1914). "The green operating room at St. Luke's Hospital." *California State Journal of Medicine*, 181–183.

Solomon, S. G., and P. Lennie (2007). "The machinery of colour vision." *Nature Reviews Neuroscience*, 8 (4): 276–286.

Seeing: Recognition, Scenes, and Patterns

Aguirre, G. K., E. Zarahn, and M. D'Esposito (1998). "An area within human ventral cortex sensitive to 'building' stimuli: Evidence and implications." *Neuron*, 21 (2): 373–383.

Bar, M. (2004). "Visual objects in context." *Nature Reviews Neuroscience,* 5 (8): 617–629.

Epstein, R. A., W. E. Parker, and A. M. Feiler (2007). "Where am I now? Distinct roles for parahippocampal and retrosplenial cortices in place recognition." *Journal of Neuroscience,* 27 (23): 6141–49.

Goldberger, A. L. (1996). "Fractals and the birth of Gothic: Reflections on the biologic basis of creativity." *Molecular Psychiatry,* 1 (2): 99–104.

O'Craven, K. M., and N. Kanwisher (2000). "Mental imagery of faces and places activates corresponding stimulus-specific brain regions." *Journal of Cognitive Neuroscience,* 12 (6): 1013–23.

Yue, X., E. A. Vessel, and I. Biederman (2006). "The neural basis of scene preferences." *NeuroReport,* 18 (6): 525–529.

Van Tonder, G. J., M. J. Lyons, and Y. Ejima (2002). "Visual structure of a Japanese Zen garden." *Nature,* 419 (6905): 359–360.

Light: Cycles and Health

Arendt, J. (2006). "Melatonin and human rhythms." *Chronobiology International,* 23 (1–2): 21–37.

Even, C., C. M. Schröder, S. Friedman, and F. Rouillon (2008). "Efficacy of light therapy in nonseasonal depression: A systematic review." *Journal of Affective Disorders,* 108 (1–2): 11–23.

O'Leary, E. S., E. R. Schoenfeld, R. G. Stevens, G. C. Kabat, K. Henderson, R. Grimson, M. D. Gammon, and M. C. Leske (2006). "Shift work, light at night, and breast cancer on Long Island, New York." *American Journal of Epidemiology,* 164 (4): 358–366.

Pandi-Perumal, S. R., V. Srinivasan, G. J. Maestroni, D. P. Cardinali, B. Poeggeler, and R. Hardeland (2006). "Melatonin: Nature's most versatile biological signal?" *Febs Journal,* 273 (13): 2813–38.

Raiten, D. J., and M. F. Picciano (2004). "Vitamin D and health in the 21st century: Bone and beyond—Executive summary." *American Journal of Clinical Nutrition,* 80 (6 Suppl): 1673S–77S.

Stevens, R. G., D. E. Blask, G. C. Brainard, J. Hansen, S. W. Lockley, I.

Provencio, M. S. Rea, and L. Reinlib (2007). "Meeting report: The role of environmental lighting and circadian disruption in cancer and other diseases." *Environmental Health Perspectives,* 115 (9): 1357–62.

Westrin, A., and R. W. Lam (2007). "Seasonal affective disorder: A clinical update." *Annals of Clinical Psychiatry,* 19 (4): 239–246.

3. SOUND AND SILENCE

Hearing and Sound

Darcy, A. E., L. E. Hancock, and E. J. Ware (2008). "A descriptive study of noise in the neonatal intensive care unit: Ambient levels and perceptions of contributing factors." *Advances in Neonatal Care,* 8 (3): 165–175.

Davis, M., D. S. Gendelman, M. D. Tischler, and P. M. Gendelman (1982). "A primary acoustic startle circuit: Lesion and stimulation studies." *Journal of Neuroscience,* 2 (6): 791–805.

Konishi, M. (1993). "Listening with two ears." *Scientific American,* 268 (4): 66–73.

Yost, W. A. (2007). "Perceiving sounds in the real world: An introduction to human complex sound perception." *Frontiers in Bioscience,* 12: 3461–67.

Music: Hearing and Healing

Cepeda, M. S., D. B. Carr, J. Lau, and H. Alvarez (2006). "Music for pain relief." *Cochrane Database of Systematic Reviews,* (2): CD004843.

Goldberger, A. L., L. A. Amaral, J. M. Hausdorff, P. Ch. Ivanov, C. K. Peng, and H. E. Stanley (2002). "Fractal dynamics in physiology: Alterations with disease and aging." *Proceedings of the National Academy of Sciences USA,* 99 (Suppl 1): 2466–72.

Grape, C., M. Sandgren, L. O. Hansson, M. Ericson, and T. Theorell (2003). "Does singing promote well-being? An empirical study of professional and amateur singers during a singing lesson." *Integrative Physiological and Behavioral Science*, 38 (1): 65–74.

Hagemann, D., S. R. Waldstein, and J. F. Thayer (2003). "Central and autonomic nervous system integration in emotion." *Brain and Cognition*, 52 (1): 79–87.

Kreutz, G., S. Bongard, S. Rohrmann, V. Hodapp, and D. Grebe (2004). "Effects of choir singing or listening on secretory immunoglobulin A, cortisol, and emotional state." *Journal of Behavioral Medicine*, 27 (6): 623–635.

Leardi, S., R. Pietroletti, G. Angeloni, S. Necozione, G. Ranalletta, and B. Del Gusto (2007). "Randomized clinical trial examining the effect of music therapy in stress response to day surgery." *British Journal of Surgery*, 94 (8): 943–947.

Levitin, D. (2006). *This Is Your Brain on Music: The Science of Human Obsession*. New York: Penguin.

Nilsson, U., N. Rawal, B. Enqvist, and M. Unosson (2003). "Analgesia following music and therapeutic suggestions in the PACU in ambulatory surgery: A randomized controlled trial." *Acta Anaesthesiologica Scandanavica*, 47 (3): 278–283.

Smith, C. A., C. T. Collins, A. M. Cyna, and C. A. Crowther (2006). "Complementary and alternative therapies for pain management in labour." *Cochrane Database of Systematic Reviews*, (4): CD003521.

Thayer, J. F., and M. L. Faith (2001). "A dynamic systems model of musically induced emotions: Physiological and self-report evidence." *Annals of the New York Academy of Sciences*, 930: 452–456.

Tracey, K. J. (2007). "Physiology and immunology of the cholinergic anti-inflammatory pathway." *Journal of Clinical Investigation*, 117 (2): 289–296.

Wago, H., and S. Kasahara (2004). "Music therapy, a future alternative intervention against diseases." *Advances in Experimental Medicine and Biology*, 546: 265–278.

Weinberger, N. M. (2004). "Music and the brain." *Scientific American*, 291 (5): 88–95.

Zatorre, R., and I. Peretz (2001). *The Biological Foundations of Music.* New York: New York Academy of Sciences.

4. COTTON WOOL AND CLOUDS OF FRANKINCENSE

Smell: Perception and Communication

Beauchamp, G. K., and K. Yamazaki (1997). "HLA and mate selection in humans: Commentary." *American Journal of Human Genetics,* 61 (3): 494–496.

DiChristina, M. (2006). "Secrets of the senses." *Scientific American,* 16 (3): 2–92.

Herz, R. (2007). *The Scent of Desire: Discovering Our Enigmatic Sense of Smell.* New York: HarperCollins.

Kodama, E., and P. Jurado (2007). "Butanone: The memory of a scent." *Journal of Neuroscience,* 27 (20): 5267–68.

McClintock, M. K. (1971). "Menstrual synchrony and suppression." *Nature,* 229 (5282): 244–245.

Porter, J., B. Craven, R. M. Khan, S. J. Chang, I. Kang, B. Judkewitz, J. Volpe, G. Settles, and N. Sobel (2007). "Mechanisms of scent-tracking in humans." *Nature Neuroscience,* 10 (1): 27–29.

Schaefer, A. T., and T. W. Margrie (2007). "Spatiotemporal representations in the olfactory system." *Trends in Neurosciences,* 30 (3): 92–100.

Schank, J. C. (2001). "Menstrual-cycle synchrony: Problems and new directions for research." *Journal of Comparative Psychology* 115 (Mar): 3–15.

Smeets, M., and P. Dalton (1999). "The nose of the beholder." *Aroma-Chology Review,* 8 (2): 1, 9–10.

Uchida, N., A. Kepecs, and Z. F. Mainen (2006). "Seeing at a glance, smelling in a whiff: Rapid forms of perceptual decision making." *Nature Reviews Neuroscience,* 7 (6): 485–491.

Smell and Healing: Essential Oils and Aromatherapy

Alford, V. (1957). "The Feast of Santiago in Galicia, 1956." *Folklore,* 68 (4): 489–495.

Cavanagh, H. M., and J. M. Wilkinson (2002). "Biological activities of lavender essential oil." *Phytotherapy Research,* 16 (4): 301–308.

Edwards-Jones, V., R. Buck, S. G. Shawcross, M. M. Dawson, and K. Dunn (2004). "The effect of essential oils on methicillin-resistant *Staphylococcus aureus* using a dressing model." *Burns,* 30 (8): 772–777.

Goel, N., H. Kim, and R. P. Lao (2005). "An olfactory stimulus modifies nighttime sleep in young men and women." *Chronobiology International,* 22 (5): 889–904.

Lusby, P. E., A. L. Coombes, and J. M. Wilkinson (2006). "A comparison of wound healing following treatment with Lavandula x allardii honey or essential oil." *Phytotherapy Research,* 20 (9): 755–757.

Masago, R., T. Matsuda, Y. Kikuchi, Y. Miyazaki, K. Iwanaga, H. Harada, and T. Katsuura (2000). "Effects of inhalation of essential oils on EEG activity and sensory evaluation." *Journal of Physiological Anthropology and Applied Human Science,* 19 (1): 35–42.

Mikhaeil, B. R., G. T. Maatooq, F. A. Badria, and M. M. Amer (2003). "Chemistry and immunomodulatory activity of frankincense oil." *Zeitschrift für Naturforschung C,* 58 (3–4): 230–238.

Touch and Massage

Alberts, J. R. (2007). "Huddling by rat pups: Ontogeny of individual and group behavior." *Developmental Psychobiology,* 49 (1): 22–32.

Beauchamp, M. S. (2005). "See me, hear me, touch me: Multisensory integration in lateral occipital-temporal cortex." *Current Opinion in Neurobiology,* 15 (2): 145–153.

Buckle, S. (2003). "Aromatherapy and massage: The evidence." *Paediatric Nursing,* 15 (6): 24–27.

Diego, M. A., T. Field, M. Hernandez-Reif, O. Deeds, A. Ascencio, and G. Begert (2007). "Preterm infant massage elicits consistent increases in vagal activity and gastric motility that are associated with greater weight gain." *Acta Paediatrica,* 96 (11): 1588–91.

Hernandez-Reif, M., G. Ironson, T. Field, J. Hurley, G. Katz, M. Diego, S. Weiss, M. A. Fletcher, S. Schanberg, C. Kuhn, and I.

Burman (2004). "Breast cancer patients have improved immune and neuroendocrine functions following massage therapy." *Journal of Psychosomatic Research,* 57 (1): 45–52.

Robinson, J., F. C. Biley, and H. Dolk (2007). "Therapeutic touch for anxiety disorders." *Cochrane Database of Systematic Reviews,* (3): CD006240.

Verhagen, A. P., C. Karels, S. M. Bierma-Zeinstra, A. Feleus, S. Dahaghin, A. Burdorf, H. C. de Vet, and B. W. Koes (2007). "Ergonomic and physiotherapeutic interventions for treating work-related complaints of the arm, neck or shoulder in adults: A Cochrane systematic review." *Europa Medicophysica,* 43 (3): 391–405.

Vollrath, M. A., K. Y. Kwan, and D. P. Corey (2007). "The micromachinery of mechanotransduction in hair cells." *Annual Review of Neuroscience,* 30: 339–365.

5. MAZES AND LABYRINTHS

Stress: Experience and Physiology

Benson, H., J. A. Herd, W. H. Morse, and R. T. Kelleher (1970). "Behaviorally induced hypertension in the squirrel monkey." *Circulation Research,* 27 (1 Suppl 1): 21–26.

Charmandari, E., C. Tsigos, and G. Chrousos (2005). "Endocrinology of the stress response." *Annual Review of Physiology,* 67: 259–284.

Goldstein, D. S. (2001). *The Autonomic Nervous System in Health and Disease.* New York: Marcel Decker.

Heijnen, C. J. (2000). "Who believes in 'communication'? The Norman Cousins Lecture, 1999." *Brain Behavior and Immunity,* 14 (1): 2–9.

McEwen, B., with E. N. Lasley. (2002). *The End of Stress as We Know It.* New York: Joseph Henry Press.

Meites, J. (1977). "The 1977 Nobel Prize in physiology or medicine." *Science,* 198 (1977): 594–596.

Nance, D. M., and V. M. Sanders (2007). "Autonomic innervation and regulation of the immune system (1987–2007)." *Brain Behavior and Immunity,* 21 (6): 736–745.

Sanders, V. M. (2006). "Interdisciplinary research: Noradrenergic regulation of adaptive immunity." *Brain Behavior and Immunity*, 20 (1): 1–8.

Sapolsky, R. M. (2004). *Why Zebras Don't Get Ulcers*. 3rd edition. New York: Holt.

Selye, H. (1976). *The Stress of Life*. New York: McGraw Hill.

Selye, H. (1998). "A syndrome produced by diverse nocuous agents. 1936." *Journal of Neuropsychiatry and Clinical Neurosciences*, 10 (2): 230–231.

Spiess, J., J. Rivier, C. Rivier, and W. Vale (1981). "Primary structure of corticotropin-releasing factor from ovine hypothalamus." *Proceedings of the National Academy of Sciences USA*, 78 (10): 6517–21.

Healing Stress: Exercise, Meditation, Tai Chi, and Yoga

Benson, H., B. A. Rosner, B. R. Marzetta, and H. P. Klemchuk (1974). "Decreased blood pressure in borderline hypertensive subjects who practiced meditation." *Journal of Chronic Diseases*, 27 (3): 163–169.

Berger, A. (2006). *Healing Pain*. Rodale.

Brown, J. D., and J. M. Siegel (1988). "Exercise as a buffer of life stress: A prospective study of adolescent health." *Health Psychology*, 7 (4): 341–353.

Dishman, R. K., H. R. Berthoud, F. W. Booth, C. W. Cotman, V. R. Edgerton, M. R. Fleshner, S. C. Gandevia, et al. (2006). "Neurobiology of exercise." *Obesity* (Silver Spring), 14 (3): 345–356.

Esch, T., J. Duckstein, J. Welke, and V. Braun (2007). "Mind/body techniques for physiological and psychological stress reduction: Stress management via Tai Chi training—A pilot study." *Medical Science Monitor*, 13 (11): CR488–497.

Fleshner, M. (2005). "Physical activity and stress resistance: Sympathetic nervous system adaptations prevent stress-induced immunosuppression." *Exercise and Sport Sciences Reviews*, 33 (3): 120–126.

Foley, T. E., and M. Fleshner (2008). "Neuroplasticity of dopamine circuits after exercise: Implications for central fatigue." *Neuromolecular Medicine*, 10 (2): 67–80.

Moraska, A., T. Deak, R. L. Spencer, D. Roth, and M. Fleshner (2000). "Treadmill running produces both positive and negative physiological adaptations in Sprague-Dawley rats." *American Journal of Physiology-Regulatory Integrative and Comparative Physiology,* 279 (4): R1321–29.

Wallace, R. K. (1970). "Physiological effects of transcendental meditation." *Science,* 167 (926): 1751–54.

West, J., C. Otte, K. Geher, J. Johnson, and D. C. Mohr (2004). "Effects of Hatha yoga and African dance on perceived stress, affect, and salivary cortisol." *Annals of Behavioral Medicine,* 28 (2): 114–118.

Yeh, G. Y., M. J. Wood, B. H. Lorell, L. W. Stevenson, D. M. Eisenberg, P. M. Wayne, A. L. Goldberger, R. B. Davis, and R. S. Phillips (2004). "Effects of tai chi mind-body movement therapy on functional status and exercise capacity in patients with chronic heart failure: A randomized controlled trial." *American Journal of Medicine,* 117 (8): 541–548.

Labyrinths and Mazes

Artress, L. (1995). *Walking a Sacred Path: Rediscovering the Labyrinth as a Spiritual Tool.* New York: Riverhead.

Hogg, S. (1996). "A review of the validity and variability of the elevated plus-maze as an animal model of anxiety." *Pharmacology Biochemistry and Behavior,* 54 (1): 21–30.

Kern, H. (2000). *Through the Labyrinth.* New York: Prestel.

Ketley-Laporte, J., and O. Ketley-Laporte (1997). *Chartres: Le Labyrinthe Déchiffré.* Jouve, Mayenne: J.-M. Garnier.

Rowling, J. K. (2000). *Harry Potter and the Goblet of Fire.* New York: Scholastic.

6. FINDING YOUR WAY . . .

Etienne, A. S., and K. J. Jeffery (2004). "Path integration in mammals." *Hippocampus,* 14 (2): 180–192.

Gabler, N. (2006). *Walt Disney: The Triumph of the American Imagination*. New York: Knopf.

Hench, J., with P. Van Pelt (2003). *Designing Disney: Imagineering and the Art of the Show*. New York: Disney Editions.

Henriques, D. Y., and J. F. Soechting (2005). "Approaches to the study of haptic sensing." *Journal of Neurophysiology*, 93 (6): 3036–43.

Menzel, R., R. J. De Marco, and U. Greggers (2006). "Spatial memory, navigation and dance behaviour in *Apis mellifera*." *Journal of Comparative Physiology A-Neuroethology, Sensory, Neural, and Behavioral Physiology*, 192 (9): 889–903.

Sternberg, E. M., and M. A. Wilson (2006). "Neuroscience and architecture: Seeking common ground." *Cell*, 127 (2): 239–242.

7. . . . AND LOSING IT

Memory

Corkin, S. (2002). "What's new with the amnesic patient H.M.?" *Nature Reviews Neuroscience*, 3 (2): 153–160.

Kandel, E. (2006). *In Search of Memory*. New York: Norton.

Milner, B. (2005). "The medial temporal-lobe amnesic syndrome." *Psychiatric Clinics of North America*, 28 (3): 599–611.

Moscovitch, M., L. Nadel, G. Winocur, A. Gilboa, and R. S. Rosenbaum (2006). "The cognitive neuroscience of remote episodic, semantic and spatial memory." *Current Opinion in Neurobiology*, 16 (2): 179–190.

Rizk-Jackson, A. M., S. F. Acevedo, D. Inman, D. Howieson, T. S. Benice, and J. Raber (2006). "Effects of sex on object recognition and spatial navigation in humans." *Behavioural Brain Research*, 173 (2): 181–190.

Squire, L. R., and P. J. Bayley (2007). "The neuroscience of remote memory." *Current Opinion in Neurobiology*, 17 (2): 185–196.

Sternberg, E. M. (2001). "Piecing together a puzzling world." *Science*, 292 (5522): 1661–62.

Alzheimer's, Inflammation, and Exercise

Heneka, M. T., and M. K. O'Banion (2007). "Inflammatory processes in Alzheimer's disease." *Journal of Neuroimmunology,* 184 (1–2): 69–91.

Perry, V. H., C. Cunningham, and C. Holmes (2007). "Systemic infections and inflammation affect chronic neurodegeneration." *Nature Reviews Immunology,* 7 (2): 161–167.

Van Praag, H., B. R. Christie, T. J. Sejnowski, and F. H. Gage (1999). "Running enhances neurogenesis, learning, and long-term potentiation in mice." *Proceedings of the National Academy of Sciences USA,* 96 (23): 13427–31.

Linking the Brain and the Immune System

Barrientos, R. M., E. A. Higgins, D. B. Sprunger, L. R. Watkins, J. W. Rudy, and S. F. Maier (2002). "Memory for context is impaired by a post context exposure injection of interleukin-1 beta into dorsal hippocampus." *Behavioural Brain Research,* 134 (1–2): 291–298.

Berkenbosch, F., J. van Oers, A. del Rey, F. Tilders, and H. Besedovsky (1987). "Corticotropin-releasing factor-producing neurons in the rat activated by interleukin-1." *Science,* 238 (4826): 524–526.

Dantzer, R., J. C. O'Connor, G. G. Freund, R. W. Johnson, and K. W. Kelley (2008). "From inflammation to sickness and depression: When the immune system subjugates the brain." *Nature Reviews Neuroscience,* 9 (1): 46–56.

Depino, A. M., M. Alonso, C. Ferrari, A. del Rey, D. Anthony, H. Besedovsky, J. H. Medina, and F. Pitossi (2004). "Learning modulation by endogenous hippocampal IL-1: Blockade of endogenous IL-1 facilitates memory formation." *Hippocampus,* 14 (4): 526–535.

Goehler, L. E., R. P. Gaykema, K. T. Nguyen, J. E. Lee, F. J. Tilders, S. F. Maier, and L. R. Watkins (1999). "Interleukin-1 beta in immune cells of the abdominal vagus nerve: A link between the immune and nervous systems?" *Journal of Neuroscience,* 19 (7): 2799–806.

Layé, S., R. M. Bluthé, S. Kent, C. Combe, C. Médina, P. Parnet, K. Kelley, and R. Dantzer (1995). "Subdiaphragmatic vagotomy blocks induction of IL-1 beta mRNA in mice brain in response to peripheral LPS." *American Journal of Physiology,* 268 (5, pt. 2): R1327–31.

Marques-Deak, A., and E. M. Sternberg (2005). "Brain-immune interactions and disease susceptibility." *Molecular Psychiatry,* 1–12.

Schneider, H., F. Pitossi, D. Balschun, A. Wagner, A. del Rey, and H. O. Besedovsky (1998). "A neuromodulatory role of interleukin-1 beta in the hippocampus." *Proceedings of the National Academy of Sciences USA,* 95 (13): 7778–83.

Wan, W., L. Wetmore, C. M. Sorensen, A. H. Greenberg, and D. M. Nance (1994). "Neural and biochemical mediators of endotoxin and stress-induced c-fos expression in the rat brain." *Brain Research Bulletin,* 34 (1): 7–14.

Watkins, L. R., M. R. Hutchinson, A. Ledeboer, J. Wieseler-Frank, E. D. Milligan, and S. F. Maier (2007). "Norman Cousins Lecture: Glia as the 'bad guys'—Implications for improving clinical pain control and the clinical utility of opioids." *Brain Behavior and Immunity,* 21 (2): 131–146.

8. HEALING THOUGHT AND HEALING PRAYER

Meditation

Barinaga, M. (2003). "Buddhism and neuroscience: Studying the well-trained mind." *Science,* 302 (5642): 44–46.

Brefczynski-Lewis, J. A., A. Lutz, H. S. Schaefer, D. B. Levinson, and R. J. Davidson (2007). "Neural correlates of attentional expertise in long-term meditation practitioners." *Proceedings of the National Academy of Sciences USA,* 104 (27): 11483–88.

Dalai Lama, H.H.T. (2002). *How to Practice the Way to a Meaningful Life.* New York: Pokey Books.

Dalai Lama, H.H.T. (2005). *The Universe in a Single Atom.* New York: Doubleday Broadway.

Davidson, R. J., J. Kabat-Zinn, J. Schumacher, M. Rosenkranz, D.

Muller, S. F. Santorelli, F. Urbanowski, A. Harrington, K. Bonus, and J. F. Sheridan (2003). "Alterations in brain and immune function produced by mindfulness meditation." *Psychosomatic Medicine,* 65 (4): 564–570.

Geirland, J. (2006). "Buddha on the Brain." Wired, 14: 1–4.

Lutz, A., L. L. Greischar, N. B. Rawlings, M. Ricard, and R. J. Davidson (2004). "Long-term meditators self-induce high-amplitude gamma synchrony during mental practice." *Proceedings of the National Academy of Sciences USA,* 101 (46): 16369–73.

Lutz, A., H. A. Slagter, J. D. Dunne, and R. J. Davidson (2008). "Attention regulation and monitoring in meditation." *Trends in Cognitive Sciences,* 12 (4): 163–169.

Melloni, L., C. Molina, M. Pena, D. Torres, W. Singer, and E. Rodriguez (2007). "Synchronization of neural activity across cortical areas correlates with conscious perception." *Journal of Neuroscience,* 27 (11): 2858–65.

Ospina, M. B., K. Bond, M. Karkhaneh, L. Tjosvold, B. Vandermeer, Y. Liang, L. Bialy, N. Hooton, N. Buscemi, D. M. Dryden, and T. P. Klassen (2007). "Meditation practices for health: State of the research." University of Alberta Evidence-Based Practice Center, Edmonton, Alberta, Canada, for the Agency for Healthcare Research and Quality. Evidence Report / Technology Assessment Number 155, AHRQ Publication no. 07-E010. Rockville, Md.

Sternberg, E. M. (2006). "A Compassionate Universe?" Review of *The Universe in a Single Atom,* by the XIV Dalai Lama, Tenzin Gyatso. *Science,* 311 (5761): 611–612.

Religious Experience and Prayer

Azari, N. P., J. Nickel, G. Wunderlich, M. Niedeggen, H. Hefter, L. Tellamen, H. Herzog, P. Stoerig, D. Birnbacher, and R. J. Seitz (2001). "Neural correlates of religious experience." *European Journal of Neuroscience,* 13 (8): 1649–52.

Beauregard, M., and V. Paquette (2006). "Neural correlates of a mystical experience in Carmelite nuns." *Neuroscience Letters*, 405 (3): 186–190.

Bély, J.-P. (2001). "Rapport médico-spirituel sur la guérison." Bureau Médical et Comité Médical International de Lourdes. February.

Borg, J., B. Andrée, H. Soderstrom, and L. Farde (2003). "The serotonin system and spiritual experiences." *American Journal of Psychiatry*, 160 (11): 1965–69.

Carrel, A. (1950). *The Voyage to Lourdes*. New York: HarperCollins.

Charcot, J. M. (1893). "Revue des maladies nerveuses et mentales." *Archives de Neurologie*, 25: 72–87.

Harris, R. (1999). *Lourdes: Body and Spirit in the Secular Age*. New York: Penguin.

Mangiapan, T. (1994). *Les Guérisons de Lourdes*. Italy: Oeuvre de la Grotte.

Taber, K. H., and R. A. Hurley (2007). "Neuroimaging in schizophrenia: Misattributions and religious delusions." *Journal of Neuropsychiatry and Clinical Neurosciences*, 19 (1): 1–4.

9. HORMONES OF HOPE AND HEALING

Placebo Effect

Finniss, D. G., and F. Benedetti (2005). "Mechanisms of the placebo response and their impact on clinical trials and clinical practice." *Pain*, 114 (1–2): 3–6.

Fuente-Fernández, R. de la, M. Schulzer, and A. J. Stoessl (2004). "Placebo mechanisms and reward circuitry: Clues from Parkinson's disease." *Biological Psychiatry*, 56 (2): 67–71.

Harrington, A. (2008). *The Cure Within: A History of Mind-Body Medicine*. New York: Norton.

Levine, J. D., N. C. Gordon, and H. L. Fields (1978). "The mechanism of placebo analgesia." *Lancet*, 2 (8091): 654–657.

Levine, J. D., N. C. Gordon, and H. L. Fields (1979). "Naloxone dose dependently produces analgesia and hyperalgesia in postoperative pain." *Nature*, 278 (5706): 740–741.

Wager, T. D., J. K. Rilling, E. E. Smith, A. Sokolik, K. L. Casey, R. J. Davidson, S. M. Kosslyn, R. M. Rose, and J. D. Cohen (2004). "Placebo-induced changes in FMRI in the anticipation and experience of pain." *Science,* 303 (5661): 1162–67.

Zubieta, J. K., Y. R. Smith, J. A. Bueller, Y. Xu, M. R. Kilbourn, D. M. Jewett, C. R. Meyer, R. A. Koeppe, and C. S. Stohler (2001). "Regional mu opioid receptor regulation of sensory and affective dimensions of pain." *Science,* 293 (5528): 311–315.

Reward and Conditioning

Ader, R., and N. Cohen (1982). "Behaviorally conditioned immunosuppression and murine systemic lupus erythematosus." *Science,* 215 (4539): 1534–36.

Bardo, M. T., and R. A. Bevins (2000). "Conditioned place preference: What does it add to our preclinical understanding of drug reward?" *Psychopharmacology* (Berlin), 153 (1): 31–43.

Exton, M. S., C. Gierse, B. Meier, M. Mosen, Y. Xie, S. Frede, M. U. Goebel, V. Limmroth, and M. Schedlowski (2002). "Behaviorally conditioned immunosuppression in the rat is regulated via noradrenaline and beta-adrenoceptors." *Journal of Neuroimmunology,* 131 (1–2): 21–30.

Goebel, M. U., A. E. Trebst, J. Steiner, Y. F. Xie, M. S. Exton, S. Frede, A. E. Canbay, M. C. Michel, U. Heeman, and M. Schedlowski (2002). "Behavioral conditioning of immunosuppression is possible in humans." *FASEB Journal,* 16 (14): 1869–73.

Hormones and Inflammation: Discovering the Link

Hench, P. S., E. C. Kendall, C. H. Slocumb, and H. F. Polley (1949). "The effect of a hormone of the adrenal cortex (17-hydroxy-11-dehydrocorticosterone: Compound E) and of pituitary adrenocorticotropic hormone on rheumatoid arthritis: Preliminary report." *Proceedings of the Staff Meetings of the Mayo Clinic, Rochester, Minnesota,* 24 (8): 181–197.

Lantz, J. (2000). "Historical profiles of Mayo Clinic: The 1950 Nobel Prize in physiology or medicine." *Mayo Clinic Proceedings,* 24.

Sex, Love, and Bonding: Neurobiological and Hormonal Bases

Carter, C. S. (1998). "Neuroendocrine perspectives on social attachment and love." *Psychoneuroendocrinology,* 23 (8): 779–818.

Insel, T. R., and L. E. Shapiro (1992). "Oxytocin receptor distribution reflects social organization in monogamous and polygamous voles." *Proceedings of the National Academy of Sciences USA,* 89 (13): 5981–85.

Kosfeld, M., M. Heinrichs, P. J. Zak, U. Fischbacher, and E. Fehr (2005). "Oxytocin increases trust in humans." *Nature,* 435 (7042): 673–676.

Mong, J. A., and D. W. Pfaff (2004). "Hormonal symphony: Steroid orchestration of gene modules for sociosexual behaviors." *Molecular Psychiatry,* 9 (6): 550–556.

Porges, S. W. (1998). "Love: An emergent property of the mammalian autonomic nervous system." *Psychoneuroendocrinology,* 23 (8): 837–861.

Winslow, J. T., N. Hastings, C. S. Carter, C. R. Harbaugh, and T. R. Insel (1993). "A role for central vasopressin in pair bonding in monogamous prairie voles." *Nature,* 365 (6446): 545–548.

Healing Hormones, Healing Emotions:
Bolstering Immunity and Health

Cutolo, M., R. H. Straub, and J. W. Bijlsma (2007). "Neuroendocrine-immune interactions in synovitis." *Nature Clinical Practice in Rheumatology,* 3 (11): 627–634.

Marques-Deak, A., and E. M. Sternberg (2007). "The biology of positive emotions." In Stephen G. Post, ed., *The Science of Altruism and Health: Is It Good to Be Good?* Oxford: Oxford University Press.

Murphy, E., and K. S. Korach (2006). "Actions of estrogen and estrogen receptors in nonclassical target tissues." *Ernst Schering Foundation Symposium Proceedings*, (1): 13–24.

Orbach, H., and Y. Shoenfeld (2007). "Hyperprolactinemia and autoimmune diseases." *Autoimmunity Reviews*, 6 (8): 537–542.

Pace, T. W. W., L. T. Negi, D. D. Adame, S. P. Cole, T. I. Sivilli, T. D. Brown, M. J. Issa, and C. L. Raison (2009). "Effect of compassion meditation on neuroendocrine, innate immune and behavioral responses to psychosocial stress. *Psychoneuroendocrinology*, 34: 87–98.

Post, S. (2007). *Altruism and Health: Is It Good to Be Good?* New York: Oxford University Press.

Post, S., and J. Neimark (2008). *Why Good Things Happen to Good People: How to Live a Longer, Healthier, Happier Life by the Simple Act of Giving.* New York: Broadway Books.

Sternberg, E. M. (2001). *The Balance Within: The Science Connecting Health and Emotions.* New York: Holt, Times Imprint.

Sternberg, E. M. (2006). "Neural regulation of innate immunity: A coordinated non-specific host response to pathogens." *Nature Reviews Immunology*, 6 (4): 318–328.

Straub, R. H. (2007). "The complex role of estrogens in inflammation." *Endocrine Reviews*, 28 (5): 521–574.

Walker, S. E., and J. D. Jacobson (2000). "Roles of prolactin and gonadotropin-releasing hormone in rheumatic diseases." *Rheumatic Disease Clinics of North America*, 26 (4): 713–736.

10. Hospitals and Well-Being

Healing Architecture: Design Based on Evidence

Beauchemin, K. M., and P. Hays (1996). "Sunny hospital rooms expedite recovery from severe and refractory depressions." *Journal of Affective Disorders*, 40 (1–2): 49–51.

Berry, L. L., D. Parker, R. C. Coile, D. K. Hamilton, D. D. O'Neill, and B. L. Sadler (2004). "The business case for better buildings." *Healthcare Financial Management*, 58 (11): 76–78, 80, 82–84.

Devlin, A. S., and A. B. Arneill. (2003). "Health care environments and patient outcomes: A review of the literature." *Environment and Behavior*, 35: 665–694.

Grossman, J. H. (2004). Putting it all together: The building blocks to create the 21st-century health care delivery system. Presentation for the Robert Wood Johnson Foundation, March, 1–24.

Kellert, S. R., J. Heerwagen, and M. Mador (2008). *Biophilic Design: The Theory, Science and Practice of Bringing Buildings to Life*. New York: John Wiley.

Malcolm, C. (2006). "Re-thinking environments for healthcare: A conversation with Derek Parker." Issue entitled *The Potential of Place*, in *See* (Herman Miller, Inc.), 4: 58–78.

Mitka, M. (2001). "Home modifications to make older lives easier." *Journal of the American Medical Association*, 286 (14): 1699–1700.

Nelson, C., T. West, and C. Goodman (2005). "The hospital built environment: What role might funders of health services research play?" Report prepared by the Lewin Group, Inc. (Contract no. 290-04-0011) for the Agency for Healthcare Research and Quality, Rockville, Md.

Stefl, M. E. (2001). "To err is human: Building a safer health system in 1999." *Frontiers of Health Services Management*, 18 (1): 1–2.

Stichler, J. F. (2001). "Creating healing environments in critical care units." *Critical Care Nursing Quarterly*, 24 (3): 1–20.

Voelker, R. (2001). "'Pebbles' cast ripples in healthcare design." *Journal of the American Medical Association*, 286 (14): 1701–702.

Zeisel, J., N. M. Silverstein, J. Hyde, S. Levkoff, M. P. Lawton, and W. Holmes (2003). "Environmental correlates to behavioral health outcomes in Alzheimer's special care units." *The Gerontologist*, 43: 697–711.

Zeisel, J. (2006). *Inquiry by Design: Environment / Behavior / Neuroscience in Architecture, Interiors, Landscape and Planning*. New York: Norton.

Hospital History: Defeating Infection, Bringing Light

Adams, A. (2008). *Medicine by Design: The Architect and the Modern Hospital, 1893–1943*. Minneapolis: University of Minnesota Press.

Campbell, M. (2005). "What tuberculosis did for modernism: The influence of a curative environment on modernist design and architecture." *Medical History,* 49 (4): 463–488.

Cook, G. C. (2002). "Henry Currey Friba (1820–1900): Leading Victorian hospital architect, and early exponent of the 'pavilion principle.'" *Postgraduate Medical Journal,* 78 (920): 352–359.

Dunn, P. M. (2007). "Oliver Wendell Holmes (1809–1894) and his essay on puerperal fever." *Archives of Disease in Childhood Fetal and Neonatal Edition,* 92 (4): F325–327.

Gill, C. J., and G. C. Gill (2005). "Nightingale in Scutari: Her legacy reexamined." *Clinical Infectious Diseases,* 40: 1799–805.

Lister, J. (1867). "On the antiseptic principle in the practice of surgery." *British Medical Journal,* 2 (September 21): 9–12.

Pittet, D., and J. M. Boyce. (2001). "Hand hygiene and patient care: Pursuing the Semmelweis legacy." *Lancet Infectious Diseases* (April): 9–20.

Taverniti, L., and A. Di Carlo (1998). "The first 'rules' of an ancient dermatologic hospital, the S. Gallicano Institute in Rome (1725)." *International Journal of Dermatology,* 37 (2): 150–155.

Tomes, N. (1994). *The Art of Asylum-Keeping: Thomas Story Kirkbride and the Origins of American Psychiatry.* Cambridge: Cambridge University Press.

Yanni, C. (2007). *The Architecture of Madness: Insane Asylums in the United States.* Minneapolis: University of Minnesota Press.

Stress and Immunity

Cohen, S., W. J. Doyle, D. P. Skoner, B. S. Rabin, and J. M. Gwaltney Jr. (1997). "Social ties and susceptibility to the common cold." *Journal of the American Medical Association,* 277 (24): 1940–44.

Cohen, S., D. Janicki-Deverts, and G. E. Miller (2007). "Psychological stress and disease." *Journal of the American Medical Association,* 298 (14): 1685–87.

Esterling, B. A., J. K. Kiecolt-Glaser, J. C. Bodnar, and R. Glaser (1994). "Chronic stress, social support, and persistent alterations in the natural killer cell response to cytokines in older adults." *Health Psychology,* 13 (4): 291–298.

Glaser, R., and J. K. Kiecolt-Glaser (2005). "Stress-induced immune dysfunction: Implications for health." *Nature Reviews Immunology,* 5 (3): 243–251.

Reichsman, F., G. L. Engel, V. Harway, and S. Escalona (1957). "Monica, an infant with gastric fistula and depression: An interim report on her development to the age four years." *Psychiatric Research Reports American Psychiatric Association,* 8: 12–27.

Healthcare Design: Cutting-Edge Creativity and New Technologies

Cizza, G., A. H. Marques, F. Eskandari, S. Torvik, M. N. Silverman, I. C. Christie, T. M. Phillips, and E. M. Sternberg (2008). "Elevated neuroimmune biomarkers in sweat patches and plasma of premenopausal women with major depressive disorder in remission." *Biological Psychiatry,* 64 (10): 907–911.

DeFanti, T. A., G. Dawe, D. J. Sandin, J. P. Schulze, P. Otto, J. Girardo, F. Kuester, L. Smarr, and R. Rao (2009). "The StarCAVE, a third-generation CAVE and virtual reality OptIPortal." *Future Generation Computer Systems,* 25 (2): 169–178.

Demetrios, E. (2001). *An Eames Primer.* New York: Universe Publishing.

Edelstein, E. A., K. Gramann, J. Schulze, et al. (2008). "Neural responses during navigation in the virtual aided design laboratory: Brain dynamics of orientation in architecturally ambiguous space." In S. Haq, C. Holscher, and S. Torgrude, eds., *Movement and Orientation in Built Environments: Evaluating Design Rationale and User Cognition.* SFB/TR 8 Report no. 015–05/2008. Report Series of the Transregional Collaborative Research Center SFB/TR 8 Spatial Cognition.

Glover, J., S. Thrun, and J. T. Matthews (2004). "Learning user models of mobility-related activities through instrumented walking aids." *Robotics and Automation, Proceedings, ICRA '04, 2004 IEEE International Conference,* 4: 3306–12.

Mendez, M. F., M. M. Cherrier, and R. S. Meadows (1996). "Depth perception in Alzheimer's disease." *Perceptual and Motor Skills*, 83 (3, pt. 1): 987–995.

Parsons, T. D., and A. A. Rizzo (2008). "Affective outcomes of virtual-reality exposure therapy for anxiety and specific phobias: A meta-analysis." *Journal of Behavior Therapy and Experimental Psychiatry*, 39: 250–261.

Tarr, M. J., and W. H. Warren (2002). "Virtual reality in behavioral neuroscience and beyond." *Nature Neuroscience*, 5 (Suppl): 1089–92.

11. Healing Cities, Healing World

The Urban Penalty: Health Costs of City Living

Haines, M. R. (1977). "Mortality in nineteenth century America: Estimates from New York and Pennsylvania census data, 1865 and 1900." *Demography*, 14 (3): 311–331.

Heidorn, K. (1979). "A chronology of important events in the history of air pollution meteorology to 1970." *American Meteorological Society*, 59 (12): 1589–97.

Morgan, W. J., E. F. Crain, R. S. Gruchalla, G. T. O'Connor, M. Kattan, R. Evans III, J. Stout, et al. (2004). "Results of a home-based environmental intervention among urban children with asthma." *New England Journal of Medicine*, 351 (11): 1068–80.

Mumford, Lewis (1938). *The Culture of Cities.* New York: Harcourt, Brace.

Picard, L. (2005). *Victorian London: The Tale of a City, 1840–1870.* New York: Weidenfeld and Nicolson.

Stone, R. (2002). "Air pollution: Counting the cost of London's killer smog." *Science*, 298 (5601): 2106–107.

Wright, R. J., H. Mitchell, C. M. Visness, S. Cohen, J. Stout, R. Evans, and D. Gold (2004). "Community violence and asthma morbidity: The Inner-City Asthma Study." *American Journal of Public Health*, 94: 625–632.

Something in the Water: Cholera Epidemiology in London, 1854

Brody, H., M. R. Rip, P. Vinten-Johansen, N. Paneth, and S. Rachman (2000). "Map-making and myth-making in Broad Street: The London cholera epidemic, 1854." *Lancet*, 356 (9223): 64–68.

Johnson, S. (2006). *The Ghost Map.* New York: Riverhead Books.

Lilienfeld, D. E. (2000). "John Snow: The first hired gun?" *American Journal of Epidemiology,* 152 (1): 4–9.

McLeod, K. S. (2000). "Our sense of Snow: The myth of John Snow in medical geography." *Social Science and Medicine,* 50 (7–8): 923–935.

Paneth, N., P. Vinten-Johansen, H. Brody, and M. Rip (1998). "A rivalry of foulness: Official and unofficial investigations of the London cholera epidemic of 1854." *American Journal of Public Health,* 88 (10): 1545–53.

Snow, J. (1854). "The cholera near Golden Square, and at Deptford." *Medical Times and Gazette,* 9: 321–322.

The Urban Advantage: Physical Activity Defeating Obesity Epidemic

Centers for Disease Control (2006). "State-specific prevalence of obesity among adults: United States." *Morbidity and Mortality Weekly Report,* 55 (36): 985–988.

Eid, J., H. G. Overman, D. Puga, and M. A. Turner (2008). "Fat City: Questioning the relationship between urban sprawl and obesity." *Journal of Urban Economics,* 63 (2): 385–404.

Ewing, R., R. C. Brownson, and D. Berrigan (2006). "Relationship between urban sprawl and weight of United States youth." *American Journal of Preventive Medicine,* 31 (6): 464–474.

Frank, L. D., M. A. Andresen, and T. L. Schmid (2004). "Obesity relationships with community design, physical activity, and time spent in cars." *American Journal of Preventive Medicine,* 27 (2): 87–96.

Hedley, A. H., C. Ogden, C. L. Johnson, M. D. Carroll, L. R. Curtin, and K. M. Flegal (2004). "Prevalence of overweight and obesity among U.S. children, adolescents and adults, 1999–2002." *Journal of the American Medical Association,* 291 (23): 2847–2850.

Lopez, R. P., and H. P. Hynes (2006). "Obesity, physical activity, and the urban environment: Public health research needs." *Environmental Health,* 5: 25.

Simonsick, E. M., J. M. Guralnik, S. Volpato, J. Balfour, and L. P. Fried

(2005). "Just get out the door! Importance of walking outside the home for maintaining mobility: Findings from the Women's Health and Aging Study." *Journal of American Geriatrics Society,* 53 (2): 198–203.

Thompson, C. (2007). "Why New Yorkers last longer." *New York Magazine,* August 12, 2007.

Vlahov, D., S. Galea, and N. Freudenberg (2005). "The urban health 'advantage.'" *Journal of Urban Health,* 82 (1): 1–4.

Designing Healthier Cities

Caracci, G. (2008). "General concepts of the relationship between urban areas and mental health." *Current Opinion in Psychiatry,* 21 (4): 385–390.

Cervero, R., and M. Duncan (2003). "Walking, bicycling, and urban landscapes: Evidence from the San Francisco Bay Area." *American Journal of Public Health,* 93 (9): 1478–83.

Dannenberg, A. L., R. J. Jackson, H. Frumkin, R. A. Schieber, M. Pratt, C. Kochtitzky, and H. H. Tilson (2003). "The impact of community design and land-use choices on public health: A scientific research agenda." *American Journal of Public Health,* 93 (9): 1500–1508.

Handy, S. L., M. G. Boarnet, R. Ewing, and R. E. Killingsworth (2002). "How the built environment affects physical activity: Views from urban planning." *American Journal of Preventive Medicine,* 23 (2 Suppl): 64–73.

Kuo, F. E. (2001). "Coping with poverty: Impacts of environment and attention in the inner city," *Environment and Behavior,* 33 (1): 5–34.

Saelens, B. E., J. F. Sallis, J. B. Black, and D. Chen (2003). "Neighborhood-based differences in physical activity: An environment scale evaluation." *American Journal of Public Health,* 93 (9): 1552–58.

Ward, S. (2004). "A framework for incorporating the prevention of Lyme disease transmission into the landscape planning and design process." *Landscape and Urban Planning,* 66: 91–106.

Zimring, C., A. Joseph, G. L. Nicoll, and S. Tsepas (2005). "Influences of building design and site design on physical activity: Research and intervention opportunities." *American Journal of Preventive Medicine,* 28 (2 Suppl 2): 186–93.

Climate Change and Disease

Bernstein, L., P. Bosch, O. Canziani, Z. Chen, R. Christ, O. Davidson, et al. (2007). *Intergovernmental Panel on Climate Change: Fourth Assesment Report.* Prepared for COP-13: 23.

Colwell, R. R. (2004). "Infectious disease and environment: Cholera as a paradigm for waterborne disease." *International Microbiology,* 7 (4): 285–289.

Crutzen, P. (2004). "New directions: The growing urban heat and pollution 'island' effect—Impact on chemistry and climate." *Atmospheric Environment,* 38: 3539–40.

Duchin, J. S., F. T. Koster, C. J. Peters, G. L. Simpson, B. Tempest, S. R. Zaki, T. G. Ksiazek, et al. (1994). "Hantavirus pulmonary syndrome: A clinical description of 17 patients with a newly recognized disease (the Hantavirus Study Group)." *New England Journal of Medicine,* 330 (14): 949–955.

Githeko, A. K., S. W. Lindsay, U. E. Confalonieri, and J. A. Patz (2000). "Climate change and vector-borne diseases: A regional analysis." *Bulletin of the World Health Organization,* 78 (9): 1136–47.

Hansen, J., L. Nazarenko, R. Ruedy, M. Sato, J. Willis, A. Del Genio, D. Koch, et al. (2005). "Earth's energy imbalance: Confirmation and implications." *Science,* 308 (5727): 1431–35.

Kerr, R. A. (2007). "Climate change: Scientists tell policymakers we're all warming the world." *Science,* 315 (5813): 754–757.

Liang, S. Y., K. J. Linthicum, and J. C. Gaydos (2002). "Climate change and the monitoring of vector-borne disease." *Journal of the American Medical Association,* 287 (17): 2286.

Lobitz, B., L. Beck, A. Hug, B. Wood, G. Fuchs, A. S. Faruque, and R. Colwell (2000). "Climate and infectious disease: Use of remote sensing for detection of *Vibrio cholerae* by indirect measurement." *Proceedings of the National Academy of Sciences USA,* 97 (4): 1438–43.

Patz, J. (2005). "Satellite remote sensing can improve chances of achieving sustainable health." *Environmental Health Perspectives,* 113 (2): A84–85.

Patz, J. A., D. Campbell-Lendrum, T. Holloway, and J. A. Foley (2005). "Impact of regional climate change on human health." *Nature,* 438 (7066): 310–317.

Staropoli, J. F. (2002). "The public health implications of global warming." *Journal of the American Medical Association,* 287 (17): 2282.

12. HEALING GARDENS AND MY PLACE OF PEACE

Frost, G. J. (2004). "The spa as a model of an optimal healing environment." *Journal of Alternative and Complementary Medicine,* 10 (Suppl 1): S85–92.

Marcus, C. B., and M. Barnes (1999). *Healing Gardens: Therapeutic Benefits.* New York: John Wiley.

Shen, Z. (2001). *Feng Shui: Harmonizing Your Inner and Outer Space.* New York: Dorling Kindersley.

Sherman, S. V. J., R. Ulrich, and V. Malcarne (2005). "Post-occupancy evaluation of healing gardens in a pediatric cancer center." *Landscape and Urban Planning,* 73: 167–183.

Stigsdotter, U. G., and P. Grahn (2003). "Experiencing a garden: A healing garden for people suffering from burnout diseases." *Journal of Therapeutic Horticulture,* 14: 38–49.

Tabacchi, M. H. (1998). "The efficacy of complementary medical treatments, as used by spas: A review of the evidence." *Alternative Therapies in Health and Medicine* (Suppl): 1–5.

Ulrich, R. (2006). "Evidence-based health-care architecture." *Lancet,* 368: S38–S39.

ACKNOWLEDGMENTS

I am grateful to the many people who provided advice and contributed their time to me during the writing of this book. Thanks to the scientists I interviewed for sharing their personal stories and their science, and to the architects whose vision of taking architecture into the realm of neuroscience is helping to start a new interdisciplinary field. I am grateful to John Eberhard, FAIA, for getting me started with his question: "How can we measure people's responses to built space?"; to Norman Koonce, FAIA, Professor Eduardo Macagno, Fred Marks, AIA, Alison Whitelaw, AIA, Dr. Eve Edelstein, and other members and associates of the Academy of Neuroscience for Architecture for their vision and advice. Special appreciation to Dr. Brenda Milner for reviewing the section on memory and H.M. Many thanks to Penny Herscovitch and Dan Gottlieb for basic training in "Architecture 101" and for their thoughtful and enthusiastic encouragement throughout the course of this project. Thanks to Dr. Donald Petzold for reviewing sections relevant to urban geography and the environment; to Aline Petzold for always helpful and encouraging feedback and for her personal insights into colorblindness. I am deeply grateful to Dr. Bernard François for sharing his original and detailed research on cases of cures at Lourdes; to Dr. Bernard François and Mme. Janine François for arranging my visit to Lourdes; and to Dr. Patrick Theillier and Archbishop Maurice Gardès for insights on medically unexplained cures at Lourdes. Thanks to Dr. Sorin Sonea, Université de Montréal, for his recollections of Hans Selye; to Dr. Mark Jackson, University of Exeter, for historical details of Hans Selye's life; and to Dr. Theodore Brown, University of Rochester, for historical expertise. Special thanks to Bruce E. Vaughn, Vice President, Disney Imagineering, for the behind-the-scenes tour of Disneyland and insights into workings of the parks; and to Bob Rogers, BRC Burbank, and Marshall Monroe, Marshall Monroe Magic, for their personal remembrances of pioneering Disney Imagineers. Thanks to Mark Dunham, President, and David Roland, Vice President, National Health Museum, and to Dr. Eric Haseltine for assistance related to Disney theme parks. Thanks to Dr. Gary Beauchamp and the Monell Chemical Senses Center faculty and staff for insights on the neuroscience of smell. Thanks to Mary Stevens, Bruce Buursma, Ruth Moen, and Joyce Bromberg for my visits to Herman Miller and Steelcase. Thanks to Ann Down for the tour of the Sun Valley meditation garden and Buddhist prayer wheel, and to Hillary Furlong and Tonia Bruess for introducing me to the labyrinth at St. Luke's Wood River Medical Center. Thanks to Carter Wormeley, GSA, for guiding me through and providing detailed historical information on St. Elizabeths Hospital, Washington, D.C. Thanks to the University of California at San Diego CalIT2 staff for the virtual reality StarCAVE demo. Thanks to Jeffrey Anderzhon, FAIA, and Eric McRoberts, AIA, for information on Waveny Care Center and assisted living design and to Dean Marek, Director, Chaplain Services, for insights on the Mayo Clinic. Thanks to Terrill Stumpf, Director, Center for Whole Health, Chicago Lights, for introducing me to the garth at Chicago's Fourth Presbyterian Church. Thanks to Dr. Valeria Rettori for sharing her personal experience of grieving. Many thanks to Dr. Orla Smith for editorial advice and feedback; to Susan Forward, Randy Goldsmith, Ann Ramsey, Cathy Runnels, and Ambassador Diana Lady Dougan for thoughtful feedback throughout the writing of this book, and to Dean and Tarja Papavassiliou for insights on Greece. Thanks to Pete Riley and Margaret Tarampi for assistance with referencing. I am grateful to my editors at Harvard University Press, Elizabeth Knoll and Maria Ascher, for their encouragement and expert advice at every stage of this project, and to Michael Fisher for persuading me to write this book.

INDEX